£18.99

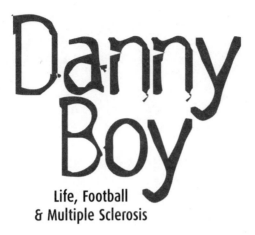

Danny Boy

Life, Football
& Multiple Sclerosis

Danny Wallace
with Kevin Brennan

highdown

Published in 2006 by Highdown,
an imprint of Raceform Ltd
Compton, Newbury, Berkshire, RG20 6NL
Raceform Ltd is a wholly-owned subsidiary of Trinity Mirror plc

A CIP catalogue record for this book is available from the British Library.

ISBN 1-905156-20-0

Designed by Tracey Scarlett

Printed in Great Britain by William Clowes Ltd, Beccles, Suffolk

CONTENTS

FOREWORD
by Sir Alex Ferguson

Danny Wallace was a crowd-pleasing footballer who could cause a buzz around the ground whenever he got the ball. It is sad to see him suffering from multiple sclerosis now and often struggling to walk, especially when I think back to how he was when I signed him for Manchester United in 1989.

But despite his illness Danny has shown character and courage to cope with his new life and I know that one of his biggest motivations has been the fact that he wants to try and help other people who might be suffering from MS or other disabilities.

When I signed Danny he was still a young man in the prime of his career after nine successful years with Southampton. I had decided that the team needed to be injected with fresh impetus and Danny was one of the players brought to the club to help us achieve that.

I know that being part of the team which won the FA Cup in his first season with United was very special to Danny, and he had a hand in setting up the crucial late equaliser for Mark Hughes in the semi-final with a great reverse pass. It was a very exciting Cup run that season because we played every tie away from home, and Danny scored a terrific goal in our match at Newcastle before setting up the winner when he beat two men and played a ball to Brian McClair. The two matches against Crystal Palace in the final were special games for everyone connected with the club, and Danny was part of the team that helped me win my first trophy as manager of Manchester United.

He had two quick feet and a turn of pace that could beat defenders. Danny offered me great speed down the flanks and could also play through the middle. He did well for us early on, but then struggled with niggling injuries and eventually left United for Birmingham.

I will always remember what a great professional he was and how exciting he could be when he was flying down the wing in full flow. I'm sure it must have been hard for him to come to terms with the loss of that speed and control because of the effects of an illness like MS. I also that know that Danny has always felt slightly upset that he didn't achieve all he had hoped for with United. But he can look back with pride on his football career and on the fact that he has battled through and come to terms with his illness after some dark times.

I will always have fond memories of him, both as a person and as a player, and I know the story of Danny's life deserves to be told.

Sir Alex Ferguson

FOREWORD
by Lawrie McMenemy

There were two things that immediately stood out when I saw Danny Wallace as a young teenager. The first was his ability as a footballer; the second was the way he seemed to be able to light up a room with that ever-present smile of his.

Danny was a lovely lad who had blistering pace and great ball control. He was also one of that rare breed, a winger who could score goals. As manager of Southampton at the time, I knew we had something a bit special on our hands when he signed for the club.

I joined Southampton in 1973 and at the time the club had virtually their pick of all the best youngsters in Hampshire, but very rarely got them from further afield. I set up a scouting system, mainly in the north-east at first, but then in the south with the help of one of the club's coaches, Bob Higgins. In many ways these efforts were the forerunners of today's modern academies which so many of the top clubs now have to help them produce and nurture good young players.

Danny was one of the kids who came through our London centre which we'd set up in Slough. When he signed apprentice forms with us in the summer of 1980, it was clear he was destined to have a big future in the game. Within months of him joining he had made his debut in the first team at the tender age of 16 in a match against the mighty Manchester United at Old Trafford. I took Danny and another youngster named Reuben Agboola along for that trip and both of them thought they were there to gain a bit of experience with the first team. However, I always intended to give them their debuts but only told them at the last minute that they were going to play in the game. It meant neither of them really had time to take it in and get nervous, and both lads went out and played brilliantly for me.

After the match the two of them joined me to be interviewed by John Motson for *Match of the Day*. After hearing my pearls of wisdom Motty wanted to know what Danny had to say about making his debut at such a tender age. The camera had to drop down about a foot and a half in order to focus on the little man, and Danny started off by referring to me as 'Lawrie'. I immediately gave him a playful clip around the ear and told him to call me 'Boss'. Danny's face broke out in that wide smile of his and I think anyone who watched the programme that night couldn't have helped but be impressed with the boy. Not just as a bright young footballer, but also as a great lad who clearly loved the game and loved life.

Those qualities never left Danny during the time I managed him and he was never really any trouble to me. He was always courteous and had a first class attitude both as an apprentice and then when he signed professional forms. He trained diligently, always gave one hundred per cent in any game he played in, scored some great goals and became a big favourite with the Southampton fans.

His record speaks for itself during his time at the Dell and as well as the contribution he made to Southampton's cause as a player, he and his younger brothers Raymond and Rodney also helped the club financially because they were all involved in transfers that eventually brought in almost £3 million to the club. All three came through the same route as youngsters and cost absolutely nothing when they signed.

There's no better feeling for a manager than to see a kid with talent make it all the way to the top, and that's what happened with Danny. He went on to play for England, and although I was no longer at Southampton when he left, I was delighted to see him get a big move to arguably the biggest club in Europe when he was transferred to Manchester United.

In more recent years it has been sad to see the onset of multiple sclerosis restricting Danny in physically doing what he would like to do. I'm sure that had the illness not struck at the time it did, Danny would have loved to have been working with youngsters as a coach or in some other capacity now, helping them to follow in his footsteps as a professional footballer.

Unfortunately that wasn't to be but the great thing is that even with MS, and after some tough times in recent years, Danny is determined to try and help other sufferers. I know that his wife Jenny and their children have been a real source of strength to him and she has been there beside him through thick and thin. It's not been an easy road for him or for them, but Danny's is a story that is worth being told.

I know that he hopes this book and the honesty with which he has written it will act as an inspiration to others and I'm sure that will be the case.

Lawrie McMenemy

PROLOGUE

THE SOUND OF SILENCE

'Danny, we've got the results of the tests we carried out on you.' My wife Jenny and I sat like two little school kids in front of the headmaster as we waited for Dr Cumming to deliver his verdict.

'It's not good news,' he continued. 'I'm afraid you have multiple sclerosis.'

I felt as though I had been hit by a sledgehammer. Those last two words of his echoed in my head as all other thoughts rushed from my mind.

I didn't say anything in reply, and neither did Jenny.

Dr Cumming tried to talk to me again, but I didn't really take any of his words in. I was trying to come to terms with the news, trying to understand how a disease like MS had managed to find its way into my body. Surely it was the sort of illness other people got? Surely it wasn't something that happened to professional footballers?

'How did I get it?' I found myself stuttering. 'What does it mean? Will I . . .'

My words trailed off as I struggled to ask the right questions. I was in shock. I knew there had been something wrong with me for a long time, and I knew it might be something serious, but I'd never drawn up a list of possible causes. Even if I had, multiple sclerosis would not have been on it. It was something I knew very little about, and because of that the diagnosis, when it was delivered, was all the more shocking.

MS had taken hold of my body, and Dr Cumming was now telling me that it would never let go. From now until the end of my life I was going to be a slave to the illness, and there was nothing I could do about it.

CHAPTER ONE

RELIEF

That meeting with Dr Cumming came at the end of a five-day stay at the Alexandra hospital in Cheadle in March 1997 during which I'd undergone all sorts of tests in order to establish to the Professional Footballers' Association's satisfaction that I had been forced to end my playing days and therefore qualified for an early pension. Those tests included a lumbar puncture – drawing spinal fluid out of my lower back through a hollow needle – and various scans, and I had a drip coming out of my arm. As well as the diagnostic tests I was also asked questions about the symptoms I had suffered and the general decline of my ability to play football and to co-ordinate properly down the right side of my body.

Well, as I said, when Dr Cumming gave Jen and I the bad news I was stunned, but, though it may sound strange to say, that feeling was soon replaced by one of overwhelming relief, because the truth was that the news suddenly explained an awful lot. It certainly helped to make the injury misery I had experienced more understandable. It provided a reason for all the niggling ailments that had plagued me during the previous few years and had forced me to become more familiar with the treatment table than the football field. From hardly ever being troubled by an injury during the entire time I played for Southampton, I had seen my career spiral downhill after a dream move in 1989 to Manchester United when I was at the peak of my game. I never fulfilled my potential at Old Trafford, and the main reason for that, as far as I was concerned, was the fact that I picked up so many injuries – nothing big, but enough to keep me out of the side for a few games just when I really needed a run of matches in the team to establish myself. Hamstrings, calf muscles, back problems – they all kept popping up on a regular basis. In many ways joining United was the beginning of the end for me, even though I could never have realised it at the time: on the day I was told I had MS, I was also informed that the first symptoms may have started some years earlier, just about the time I made the move to Old Trafford.

I joined United having made a name for myself as a goalscoring winger who had the sort of pace that always made defenders feel uncomfortable. Running fast was something that had come naturally to me since I was a young boy kicking a ball around on the streets of South London. It was never something I ever thought about or had to work on. It was second nature to me; shooting down the wing with the ball at my feet had always come easily to me. From the moment I first kicked a football I felt comfortable with the game; it was almost as if playing football was what I was meant to do with my life. There was never an ounce of doubt in my mind that I wouldn't make it. I wasn't flash about it, I was just being honest. I knew I had ability and I knew I had the dedication to take me where I wanted to go.

At the age of sixteen I was playing in the Southampton first team, and my career went from strength to strength. It all seemed pretty easy and was even more enjoyable than I could ever have imagined. I was playing football every day of my life and getting paid for it. I also began to get a lot of attention. The fans liked me, I was in the newspapers and on TV, and life was good. When you're a young professional footballer at the top of your game, you never believe anything is going to come along to spoil things. You're in a football bubble, and whatever goes on in the real world never seems to have much of an impact on you. If you are young, fit and being paid good money for doing a job most of your mates would give their right arm for, it's very difficult to get a real grip on the fact that one day it's all going to end and you will have to look for something else to do.

For most players, that day comes in their mid-thirties after two decades in the game. Some have to pack in early because of injury, and I suppose at the back of the minds of most players lurks the thought that it might happen to them, but getting something like MS never entered into my thoughts. For a start, like most people I never really had any idea what the disease was about. It was something other people got, not something you heard about in football. Broken legs, cartilage problems, knee injuries – they were the sort of things that could end a footballing career prematurely, not multiple sclerosis. Of course that kind of thinking is illogical and a bit stupid because, like any other disease, MS is indiscriminate. It doesn't matter who you are or what you do, postman, factory worker, doctor, judge, footballer. It can happen to anyone, and on that day at the Alexandra I found out that it had happened to me.

By that time I had stopped playing football simply because I wasn't physically able to carry on. I was in the team that won United's first trophy under Alex Ferguson after beating Crystal Palace in an FA Cup final replay in 1990 at Wembley. I fulfilled a boyhood dream that night when I picked up my winner's medal, and it seemed as though I was going to be part of something big. Manchester United was, and still is, a massive club. I had arrived at Old Trafford the year before for £1.2 million after over a decade with Southampton. I was 25 years old, and it seemed like the perfect move for me. But what should have been the start of the best period of my career soon began to descend into a frustrating nightmare of injury and missed opportunity. As United once again began to build a team that would dominate the English game, I found myself on the outside looking in. My form suffered, and by the spring of 1993 it was clear I was surplus to requirements as far as Fergie was concerned. In the autumn of that year I was transferred to Birmingham City, and eighteen months later I was farmed out on loan to Wycombe Wanderers. By that time the pain and fatigue I was suffering as I tried to continue as a full-time professional meant that I could hardly manage a competitive match, and less than two years after leaving one of the biggest clubs in the world I found myself trying to salvage my career by having a pre-season trial with Mansfield Town. In the end, reality forced me to admit defeat and accept the fact that I was no longer able to play the game I'd loved for as long as I could remember. I became an ex-footballer.

Life may be sweet when you're playing, but it becomes pretty scary when you have to stop. Even in normal circumstances it would have been a problem for me, because I'd done little or nothing to prepare for the day. My wife Jenny wasn't blinkered like me. She'd often asked what I was going to do when the time came to stop playing, but I'd never given her a straight answer. I had this vague idea in my head that I would like to work for my coaching badges and then maybe help bring through youngsters to the professional ranks, but I'd done nothing about it. When the end came and I knew I couldn't carry on playing I lived in limbo for months. I knew I was finished, but at the same time I didn't want to admit it to anyone else. I just slipped away from the game that had been a part of my life for so long and moped around the house. What made it seem worse was that I didn't feel ill; having stopped training on a regular basis I wasn't suffering the after-effects that had been so draining for me.

I was without a salary and, of course, still faced with the normal day-to-day costs and problems any family has, so I soon realised I had to start getting my life sorted out. I had a pension set up with the Professional Footballers' Association, but it wasn't due to mature for another couple of years. If I wanted to get my money early I was told that I needed to prove that I had been forced to pack in playing, and for that I needed to undergo a medical examination. Which is when I found myself in a room with Jenny listening to a doctor telling me I was suffering from MS.

As I said, the feeling of relief I experienced may seem an odd emotion, but in a strange way the diagnosis made me feel normal again. It didn't give me back my career, but it gave me a reason for having to stop playing. So much suddenly became clear. I hadn't been an injury-prone footballer after all; I'd been suffering from MS all along. The silly little injuries, the frequency of them, the feeling of pins and needles in my feet, having to sleep for more than sixteen hours solid after training sessions in order to be ready for the next day – now I had an explanation for it all, and because of that my predominant emotion that day was relief. I didn't exactly leave the room smiling, but I did leave it knowing I hadn't cheated anyone or taken the easy option and not played when I could have done. I'd known that all along of course, but there were some people who thought and suggested otherwise. I wasn't going to go shouting it from the rooftops, but at least I had an explanation and the picture had become clearer.

But it didn't take long for the next emotion to arrive, and that was fear, pure fear. Fear of the unknown; fear of what was going to happen to my body, my wife and my family; fear of how I would be able to function as the disease slowly but surely took over my body and made even the simplest tasks difficult; and fear of what people would think of me. Once upon a time I was Danny Wallace, professional footballer. I had become a first-team regular as a teenager, I had played for England, I had signed for Manchester United, I had been one of the fastest players around. Now people would see me losing my balance and struggling to walk; they would notice the person who used to leave top defenders struggling to keep up with him barely being able to shuffle along the pavement. It was a frightening thought. After that first diagnosis I knew little about the disease, but I did realise that my whole life was about to change.

Ironically I had done some charity work about five years earlier for Action and Research for Multiple Sclerosis, or ARMS, after meeting its chairman Anita Best. She was a sufferer herself, and at the time I was at United while Raymond and Rodney, my brothers, were both with Leeds. All three of us got involved in a series of sponsored walks between football grounds ending at Wembley on the day of the FA Cup final. The walks started in January, and I went along to Crystal Palace's Selhurst Park ground one Sunday to help lead an eight-mile walk with their manager Steve Coppell and the Wimbledon boss, Peter Withe, which ended at Millwall's ground. I saw and heard about some of the effects MS could have, but it was all at arm's length. I felt sorry for the people and was happy to be able to do something to help, but it never once crossed my mind that I might one day have to cope with it myself.

So I had the diagnosis, and that was something of a comfort after all those anxious, injury-ravaged years, but I still wasn't fully sure what the consequences might be. When it came to the details and how MS could affect you I had little idea of what it might mean for me. I was of course told about the form of the illness I had, which was the spinal variety. It meant that my nervous system would be attacked, and in my case it was the right side of my body that was suffering. The good news was that the condition wasn't life-threatening, which the other variety is. I would simply have to live with multiple sclerosis for the rest of my life, and learn to cope. It wasn't going to go away, and I was told that it might get worse. I would have problems with my hand, leg and back. Once, I had been able to run faster than most players in the First Division; now I had to get used to the prospect of shuffling along and possibly having to use a cane to help me walk. I still had a life, but it was going to have to be a re-designed life to help me cope with the illness.

As ridiculous as it may seem, when we drove away from the hospital that day I wasn't that upset or depressed. It was only when I walked through my front door and sat down that I began to think about what it would mean. The relief at knowing what was behind my problems soon began to disappear, and during the days that followed the full weight of being told I had MS slowly began to sink in.

The first thing that really hit home was the fact that I wasn't going to recover from what I had. Before all the tests I'd hoped, in the back of my mind, that whatever was troubling me would have a cure. It might be something strange and not very well known, but I thought that once the medical people got to the bottom of it they would be able to start treating me and at some stage in the future I would be back to something like my normal self. But that wasn't going to be the case, which meant I would have trouble finding any sort of job that involved physical work, and considering I was qualified for very little other than football, it meant that Jenny would have to continue to go out and earn money. By this time she had a job with the NHS helping adults with disabilities, and she also had part-time work in telesales and at British Home Stores. It was ironic that her work with the NHS should involve her with disabled people. She was doing it before I was diagnosed, and perhaps it helped her cope with the news, because she had seen people at first hand with problems far greater than anything I had.

But Jenny has since told me that despite sitting next to me looking calm and cool on the journey back from Dr Cumming after receiving the news about my MS, her mind was racing. She had gone into overdrive thinking about what it meant for us as a couple, and as a family. Before the diagnosis, she had thought I had something wrong with me that was life-threatening. She was obviously relieved to hear that that wasn't the case and that I should live to a ripe old age, but then she immediately started to go through all the possibilities of what might lie ahead for us all.

I was completely oblivious to what she was going through, and over the following months not once did I bother to actually ask her how she felt. I might have been the one with the illness, but mine wasn't the only life that would change. We were all in it together, me, Jenny and the kids, but instead of reaching out for them I slowly began to push them away. They supported me, but I gave them nothing in return, because I soon began to slip into self-centred pity and depression where I seemed to have no room for anyone else.

The truth was, I felt cheated. Cheated out of what when I was sixteen had promised to be a fine career in professional football. I'd heard people say that the reality of having to stop playing football can be a bit of a slap in the face for some players. Well, as I said, after hearing that I had MS I felt as though I'd been hit by a sledgehammer. What's more, I really wasn't sure if I was ever going to recover from the blow.

CHAPTER TWO

FOOTBALL CRAZY

I suppose that because I broke into the Southampton first team at the age of sixteen, a lot of people assumed I was a local boy. But I'm a South Londoner from Deptford – a lot closer to the Thames than the Solent – and I spent the early part of my life growing up there.

I was the sort of kid who ate, drank and breathed football, which meant that pretty much everything else in my life took a back seat, including my schoolwork. I think my attitude probably drove my poor mum and dad crazy, but at the same time they could see how I loved the game, and by the time I was ten or eleven years old they had the consolation that people who had seen me play would say that they thought I had the potential to do well. Of course there were probably thousands of kids who had the same idea, and there might have been quite a few who had as much ability, but football has a way of making sure that only a very few actually come through to make it as a professional; the others fall by the wayside for one reason or another. I knew I had ability and, looking back, even at a very young age I had the sort of dedication and determination which is vital if you are going to make it. Maybe if I'd shown the same tunnel vision when it came to my schoolwork things might have turned out differently for me, but perhaps there was something in my genes that meant I was destined to play football. After all, it wasn't just me who went on to become a professional footballer: my brothers Rodney and Raymond followed in my footsteps, and my elder brother Clive was also a decent player, although he never made his living from the game.

My mum and dad, Joan and Vincent, met in South London after travelling to England from Jamaica in the 1950s. They came over individually to start a new life and settled in the Deptford area after they married. It wasn't too long before Clive arrived on the scene, in August 1962, and around seventeen months later he got a little playmate. I was born on 21 January 1964 and named David Lloyd. For some reason I was soon referred to as Danny and the name has stuck ever since. We certainly weren't a well-off family, but both my parents worked really hard – Mum as an auxiliary nurse, and Dad as a labourer on various building sites – and did the best they could for us. I began my life in a rented flat in a run-down three-storey house in New Cross. It was a horrible place. My parents put in a lot of work trying to make it as homely and comfortable as possible, but they were always fighting a losing battle because there were rats crawling everywhere. Apparently they were there before we moved in, and they were still there when we left. The infestation was never properly dealt with, and I found it frightening. I still have a fear of rats, and it's all because of living there, even if it was only for about a year. I remember Dad setting traps all over the place, and being woken up at night as I heard them go off without being sure just how close the rats were to me. Happily, we moved into a council flat in Deptford after that, and the good thing was that the place was four storeys high and we were on the top floor. I was convinced that meant there was no way a rat would be able to get to me! It was a decent block, and I have some very happy memories of the place.

By the time England won the World Cup in the summer of 1966 I was already hooked on kicking a ball about. By all accounts I was full of energy from the time I first entered the world. Pretty soon after mastering the art of walking I began to run around all over the place, and if there was a ball at my feet I enjoyed it even more. My love of the game grew by the day. Although Clive was less than two years older than me he was still my big brother and he always looked out for me. One day, when I was about six years old, he appeared with a brand-new football as a present. It wasn't Christmas or my birthday; he'd just decided that I deserved a brand-new ball and had gone out and bought one for me. At the age of six you don't really stop to think about how your eight-year-old brother has managed to buy you a ball. You just take the gift and get on with enjoying it. Had I bothered to ask him how he got it I would have found out that he'd nicked the money from Mum's purse. Not the smartest of moves. His heart might have been in the right place, but he soon learnt that it was the wrong thing to do. Dad told him in no uncertain terms that he wasn't very happy. He got a telling-off and a whack for his trouble, but at least I got to keep the ball.

By this time my parents had another couple of mouths to feed after Mum gave birth to twins Rodney and Raymond in October 1969. At about this time I also became aware of another little boy who used to visit us in the summer and stay for the whole of the school holidays. His name was Paul and when he was introduced to me I was told by my dad, 'this is your brother.' It didn't really occur to me to ask why he wasn't around in the house all the time like my other brothers, he was a bit younger than me and I just got on with playing with him and having fun just like kids do. It wasn't until a few years later that I actually found out that Paul had been fathered by my dad with another woman who lived locally. Paul lived with his natural mother but was always welcomed at our house and my mum never had a problem with it, and he would often be around. He and his mother eventually moved from south London to Basingstoke but we still saw quite a bit of him when he came back to visit us and over the years Clive, Raymond, Rodney and me have always stayed in touch with Paul.

In the meantime, Clive and I had a great time together. We always seemed to be playing games and knocking a football around. Clive was also a very good cricketer, taking after my dad, who played to a pretty decent standard, but it was always football for me, and by the time I was eight I was beginning to take the game seriously. I played whenever I could, whether it was outside in the recreation area near our flats or at school with my mates. I hated school, even at that age; the only thing I enjoyed was sport and playing with my friends during break time. Even at primary school I couldn't wait to get home and muck about, which usually involved a football. I was really in love with the game and remember being bought a pair of Pele football boots by my parents which I slept with, because they were so special to me. When I started my secondary education, I really began to feel that I could go all the way and become a professional footballer, without being flash about it. I knew from what other people said after they had watched me play that they believed I was good at the game, and everything felt as though it came pretty easily to me. I felt very comfortable with the ball at my feet, I had a lot of pace for a kid of my age, and although I was small, I was also pretty strong.

I did suffer a bit of a set-back at around this time because of a freak injury. I was playing with Clive in the street and we were using a wooden fence to kick the ball against as part of our game. It was a windy day and on top of the fence there was a big advertising board. Suddenly a gust of wind hit the board and rocked it off its hinges. The thing came crashing down on me and hit my ankle. I was in agony and had to be helped up to our flat by Clive and his friend Michael Brown. As soon as I got there mum took a look at the injury and using all of her skills as an auxiliary nurse, started to try and ease the pain. The trouble was it only got worse, and Clive and Michael ended up having to take me to Millers Hospital in Deptford. The form of transport they used wasn't the best; because I was still pretty small they decided to stick me in a pram that the twins had used and then proceeded to rush me down to the hospital along a cobbled street as I bounced along and clung to the sides of the pram. The diagnosis from the doctor was that my ankle was broken, but he also wanted to know who had been messing about with my ankle and he clearly wasn't too impressed with what had gone on. None of us wanted to tell him that it was mum who had poked around, especially as she was a trained auxiliary nurse!

At that time, in the early to mid-1970s, there weren't too many role models for a young black kid because most teams up and down the country were almost exclusively made up of white players. The fact that black footballers were in a minority didn't bother me because I hadn't really experienced any prejudice growing up. The kids of my age where I lived all seemed to get on well together, no matter what their colour was. To be honest, I never really gave being black a second thought; I just got on with my life, and it was a contented life. I didn't watch that much football – I preferred to be out there playing – but I was a West Ham fan by the time I moved to West Greenwich school when I was eleven. Millwall were right on my doorstep, but I followed West Ham – which probably had something to do with the fact that Clyde Best, the Hammers' black forward from Bermuda, was part of the team at the time. But if he was a role model for me, it was only on a subconscious level.

By the time I got to West Greenwich they had already heard that I was a decent footballer thanks to Clive. He'd gone there a couple of years earlier and had let anyone who would listen know that his kid brother was a bit special with a football at his feet. Happily, I managed to live up to all the hype, and it wasn't long before I began playing on a regular basis for the school team. It was a good school, and I was lucky to come under the wing of a great sports teacher called Keith Hodder. He did a tremendous job with all the kids and was particularly helpful to me. I got all the encouragement I needed from him, and eventually he was instrumental in helping me to get trials with some professional clubs. He was the sort of teacher who got the best out of the kids he taught, and they wanted to do well for him. That was certainly true in my case. I enjoyed all the sport I took part in. Although football was always the number one for me, I also loved athletics. It helped that I happened to be naturally good at sprinting; I always seemed to win races like the 100 and 200 metres.

I was playing matches every week, for the school and for the district side, Blackheath, which boasted a decent team that included the likes of Paul Elliott – or 'Tat' as he was known, for some reason – and Paul Walsh, both of whom went on to play professionally. Walsh was little, just like me. There was really nothing of him, but he was very quick and very brave, with an instinct for scoring that was to be so important for him in later years. He was very tricky to mark too, and would often make opposition defenders look stupid because he could turn so well; before they were able to do anything about it, he was away, or he had managed to get a shot on goal. Paul Elliott was a pretty imposing figure even when he was a kid, a dominating defender, but the great thing about him was that he was also a very good footballer and felt perfectly at home with the ball at his feet. He had the confidence to pass the ball, not just hoof it upfield, which for someone as big as he was made him really stand out. It was a great shame when his professional career at Chelsea was cut short due to injury.

I also played for a Sunday church team in Deptford called St Paul's, and once again it was a good side. There was one kid who played up front while I was with them and always managed to score goals. He seemed a bit of a natural to everyone and I think we all thought he would make it one day as a professional. But while I went on to Southampton, this particular kid found it difficult to get a league side to take him on. He played a bit of non-league football and was eventually given a chance by Crystal Palace. The rest, as they say, is history. The player's name was Ian Wright, and he went on to become one of the most prolific goalscorers in the modern English game. We ended up playing against each other at Wembley in the 1990 FA Cup final, and although Palace came off second best after a replay, Wrighty still managed to leave his mark in the first match by coming on as a substitute and scoring two goals.

But if Keith Hodder was getting the best out of me, the other teachers at West Greenwich were struggling to do the same. To be fair to them, they never really stood a chance and were never likely to get my academic results to match up to my sporting achievements. The simple fact was that I didn't really have to work hard to be good at football, but I did when it came to my other schoolwork. I just couldn't see the point of it. I knew I was going to be a footballer and that was going to be how I earned a living, so what was the point of wasting time on other things which were no more than an unwanted distraction? At the time it made perfect sense to me, but I'm certainly not proud of the fact now. The only good grades I got were in woodwork.

Looking back now, it seems incredible that I was allowed to get away with so much at school. I'm sure Mum and Dad weren't too happy with me, but at the same time they were very supportive when it came to my football. I had a couple of trials with Millwall and Arsenal when I was about twelve, but nothing came of them, although I did train with Millwall a few times. Keith Hodder was right behind me when it came to trying to get attached to a professional club, and he obviously had enough faith in my ability to believe that it was worth my while having a trial with Southampton. They weren't exactly a local club – one of only two professional clubs in the whole of Hampshire – but they held trials at Slough that attracted a lot of kids from the London area.

As I said, the idea for me to go there came from Keith, who during a coaching course had sung my praises to John McGrath, the former Southampton defender who was still doing some work for the club. After travelling there with Keith one day and taking part in one of their sessions, I was asked to go back and start training with them on a regular basis twice a week after school. It sounded great to me, and at that age I gave no real thought as to how I was going to make the journey to Slough on a regular basis. Thankfully, Keith and the school, in the form of our headmaster Ron Dunne, came to my rescue. Every Tuesday and Thursday evening Keith would take me on the two-hour journey via under- and overground trains to Slough for training, and the school actually paid for me to do it, which was a great gesture on their part. They obviously wanted to give me as much support as they could, and I'm sure Keith was instrumental in it all.

From the moment I started training with Southampton I felt really comfortable. Although they were a First Division club (the equivalent of today's Premiership), there was a homely feel to everything and everyone. Bob Higgins, who was in charge of the youngsters at the centre in Slough, was a capable coach who looked after all the boys and made everyone feel relaxed. He seemed to be one of those coaches who was able to get the trust of the players he worked with. He hadn't been a top player, and there were no grand strategies or plans on the training field; he just coached the basics straightforwardly and simply, and went over them so that they stuck in your mind. At the same time he always tried to make the sessions fun. I don't remember being given any specialised training at the time, but there's no doubt in my mind that Bob did the right thing for boys of that age, and he brought me along at the right pace. I was lucky to have someone like him around at that stage. I think his main strength was the way he encouraged us all, and because of that we were all able to gain confidence. And there were some decent players at those sessions. It was there that I first met the likes of Reuben Agboola, who travelled from North London, and George Lawrence, who came from West London and has remained a lifelong friend.

Things went well for me personally, and by the time I was fourteen Southampton were keen to offer me schoolboy forms, which was really the next step on the ladder for any budding young footballer. The funny thing was that on the day I was supposed to sign the form, Bob Higgins turned up without the appropriate one. He actually had to go to Millwall and borrow one from them. Years later, after Keith had gone to live and coach football in the United States, he bumped into Gordon Jago who was the Millwall manager at the time, in the late 1970s. Apparently he was horrified when Keith told him the story about the form, because he realised that Millwall had missed out on signing me and I had been playing my football right on their doorstep. Even today I sometimes wonder how I ended up at The Dell when there were so many clubs closer to where I lived, Millwall first among them.

But it wasn't all football, football, football, because at about the same time as I was signing up with Southampton I started dating my first real girlfriend. Her name was Jennifer Giddings, and she lived a stone's throw away from our flat. We both used the same recreation area called the Kent that all the kids shared as a meeting place. We all seemed to get on well and everyone knew everyone else. As well as a play area there was also a hall where they would hold discos, and the kids would generally use it as a place to hang out with their mates. I'd seen Jenny around the place with some of her friends but had never done too much about talking to her. One day I decided to ask if she wanted to go and see a film with me, and she said yes. I'm not too sure why, but it didn't take long before we were seeing quite a bit of each other, even though we were only fourteen years old. Her mum and dad didn't really know we were going out together. But Jenny didn't keep it quiet because she was white and I was black; it was simply that they might have thought we were too young to be dating on such a regular basis.

Everything continued to go well on the football front as the 1970s played themselves out, and I was more convinced than ever that I was going to make it and become a professional. I was being well coached during my weekday sessions and I also got the benefit of playing for the Southampton schoolboy side against similarly aged sides from other Football League teams, not all of them First Division. These matches were usually played with just a few people watching from the sidelines, but they always felt special, mainly because I loved the idea of playing in a Southampton shirt. It gave me a taste of what things could be like for me if I managed to go all the way and become a professional footballer.

All the while I was getting physically stronger, and the training I did really helped my fitness. Our flat in Deptford played a part in the regime in those days. We didn't have a lift in the block so I would run up and down the stairs several times a day. Even going shopping with my mum did me some good because Clive and I would bound up the steps carrying heavy bags from the local supermarket – my own special form of weight training! I also got a taste of playing alongside adults, because Bob Higgins managed non-league Deal Town for a while. As a fifteen-year-old I played up front against some grisly characters who had been around the block a few times and were more than happy to dish out some physical stick to a young kid. But I more than managed to hold my own when I played. My performances even attracted some headlines in the local paper.

As I've already said, I could hardly be accused of being self-motivated when it came to most of my schoolwork, and as the time approached when I could legally leave West Greenwich I had even less incentive to work hard on the academic side of things. This was because before I left in the summer of 1980 I was offered a contract as an apprentice with Southampton, so I knew as I sat down to take my CSE exams that not only was I a matter of weeks away from leaving school for ever, I would also be playing football with a top English club as my first job. It was a dream come true for me, and I was determined to go all the way and one day play First Division football.

That day would come a lot sooner than I could ever have imagined.

CHAPTER THREE

SAINT DANNY

Lawrie McMenemy frightened me. Don't get me wrong, he wasn't a horrible man who would bawl and shout at his players. In fact he was a really nice guy and a great manager. It was simply his physical presence that I found daunting. Not only was I a kid of sixteen when I signed for Southampton, I was also quite small, and Lawrie was about a foot taller than my five feet five inches. He was a commanding figure, an ex-Guardsman. I could imagine him looking even bigger in uniform.

There was no doubt he was the boss when I arrived that summer of 1980 for my first day as an apprentice at Southampton's training ground. I had seen him before when he watched one of the schoolboy matches I was playing in for the club, but I'd never spoken to him, and the memory I had from that game was of seeing him standing by the touchline in his big dark trenchcoat talking to Bob Higgins. I'm not sure how it was decided which particular kids would eventually be taken on by the club, but I think Bob had a lot to do with it, and of course we all realised that we wouldn't be doing our chances any harm if we performed well in a game that was being watched by the club's manager. Whether that match had any bearing at all on me eventually being offered apprenticeship terms I don't really know. I don't suppose Lawrie recognised any of the new intake on that first day of training.

It was only a few weeks after I had left school, and I was so excited at the prospect of being part of the club on a full-time basis – despite being, as an apprentice, just about the lowest of the low. As well as training we were expected to do all the menial jobs around the place, things like cleaning the toilets and painting the stands at

The Dell, Southampton's compact home ground which, in spite of its small capacity, used to generate a great atmosphere. Having to do that sort of job didn't bother me; I just saw it as part of the adventure I was setting out on. For years I had dreamt of being part of a professional club and spending my days training and playing football. Now I had the chance to do just that, and as far as I was concerned I was in heaven, even if the toilets did smell a bit.

As well as marking the start of my career at Southampton, that summer also saw another forward arrive at The Dell – though this addition was a high-profile one for Lawrie's already experienced first-team squad. To everyone's surprise, the manager had announced a few months earlier that Kevin Keegan would be joining the club from Hamburg. At the time, Keegan was the European footballer of the year and one of the biggest names in the game. It was a real coup for a club like Southampton to sign someone of his stature in the game, and it showed once again that big Lawrie was capable of attracting top players. Keegan joined a squad that contained the likes of Dave Watson and Charlie George, and also some great homegrown talent like Mick Channon, who had started with the club before moving to Manchester City and had returned to The Dell in 1979, and Steve Williams, who was a real talent and went on to play for Arsenal. Of course, they were all a world away from me and my fellow apprentices, but I couldn't help getting a real buzz from the fact that I was part of the same club as them. They were players I'd only really seen on TV, and suddenly I was getting the chance to rub shoulders with them and watch them in training. It was thrilling, and I loved every minute of it.

All the apprentices had to report for pre-season training early, mainly due to the fact that we had to get everything ready for the first team when they returned after their summer break a week later. Because I lived in South London it was impossible for me to commute to Southampton, so I made my way to the stadium every day from digs the club had found for me – meaning that I stayed with a local family, Terry and Sheila Price and their kids Alison and Andrew, in their house, which was in a place called Bitterne. The deal was that you got a room and all of your meals cooked for you, which allowed the player to concentrate on his football and not worry about the basic things. It also meant that there was always someone around, and that could be a help for some of the boys if they felt a bit homesick. I wasn't sure how I would react to it all, but I settled in really well and soon got into a routine. I used to travel back to London every two or three weeks and kept my relationship going with Jenny, who would often turn up at Waterloo on a Saturday evening to meet me when I had a weekend at home. It was nice to go back to London, but if I'm honest, I think I very soon began to build myself a new life in Southampton. It was different to London and probably had a more homely feel to it, but that suited me. I think it was the same for the other lads who were taken on as apprentices. We trained hard and got on with the chores we were given without any complaints. It was just the way things were.

It also helped that the first-team players were pretty laid back. There was no great feeling of 'them' and 'us', although we certainly didn't mix on the training pitch, and off it we tended to have assigned jobs for particular players. I cleaned the boots for Charlie George and Dave Watson. Both of them treated me well and both were good tippers, especially at Christmas. It was a big help to a kid to have a player who would give you some extra cash. When I signed as an apprentice I was earning £28 per week, so having a few more pounds in my pocket now and then didn't do any harm at all. The first-team players were earning nothing like the Premiership stars of today, but they were still being paid decent money; there was no way players such as Channon, Keegan, George and Watson would have been playing for the club if they weren't being paid what they were worth. All of them were big stars who had earned their reputations over a number of years.

As I said, from the outset I was happy to be a part of this club. I enjoyed the training and the fact that my life was now all about playing football. Watching the seasoned professionals at work was a real thrill for me, and it gave all the apprentices something to aim for. We were all in the same situation: we desperately wanted to be taken on as full professionals after we'd finished our two-year apprenticeship.

It was a long road and I was just setting out on it, but I was prepared to be patient and to work hard. I knew that the best thing I could do was to keep learning and make sure that I played well with the youth team.

By the time November arrived I'd played a few games and felt I'd done pretty well. Then, at the end of the month, a couple of days before the first team were due to play Manchester United, I got some news that I thought confirmed things were moving in the right direction for me: I was told that I'd be travelling with the party for the trip to Old Trafford.

Travelling with the team was not unusual for an apprentice, although it was usually after you had been there for a year that you got the nod to be part of the set-up for a match. The idea was to give some of the kids a taste of what it was like to be in a first-team party for a big away trip. It meant that you went on the journey as a bit of a dogsbody in many ways, helping out with all the chores and making sure everything was all right for the team members, but that wasn't a problem because the experience itself was reward enough, especially if it was a game like Manchester United.

I trained with the youth team on the Thursday, and the next day I duly turned up to help load on all the kit, as the first team got ready to travel north on the coach for an overnight stay in a plush hotel. I stayed pretty quiet during the four-hour journey and sat at the front of the coach while the senior players stuck to the back and played cards. I wasn't the only youngster on board for the trip: Reuben Agboola, who was about twenty months older than me, also travelled, but he had already been taken on as a professional about six months earlier after coming through the apprentice ranks via the Slough training sessions.

When we got to our hotel I helped unload all the players' gear, then walked into the reception area, where Lawrie McMenemy was waiting for me.

'I'm going to put you in with someone who'll look after you, son,' he said. 'You'll be rooming with Mick Channon.'

Mick was great about the prospect of having to look after a kid like me, and one of the first things he did was sit me down and make a cup of tea to help calm my nerves and make me feel more at home. Silly things like this, and going for our evening meal and listening to all the banter, were new to me, and by the time we turned in at about 9.30 that night I was exhausted from all the excitement.

On the morning of the game we had our pre-match meal and set off for Old Trafford. Once again I helped to load and unload the kit, all the time thinking about going to this famous stadium for the first time and being able to watch my club play there. Then, once we'd arrived, first-team coach Lew Chatterley suggested I go out on to the Old Trafford pitch and have a good look around. The place had hardly any fans in it because there were about 90 minutes to go before kick-off, but it was still impressive, and I went back into the dressing room dreaming about the day when I would get the chance to run out on to that turf and take on United.

I sat around the visitors' dressing room for about ten minutes or so, wondering when I'd be told to leave and what sort of seat I would have to watch the game from. Then, about an hour before the match was due to start, Lawrie called me to one side and said just two words in a very matter-of-fact way.

'You're playing.'

After I got over the shock of it and made sure that he wasn't joking, I didn't really have time to dwell on the fact that I was about to make my league debut against Manchester United at Old Trafford at the age of just 16 years and 314 days, in the process becoming the youngest ever player to appear in the Southampton first team. It was a brilliant piece of man-management from Lawrie and typical of him in so many ways. I found out later that he'd always planned to give me and Reuben Agboola our debuts against United, but he waited until virtually the last minute to tell me. It meant I never had time to worry about anything; I just picked up the number seven shirt of Kevin Keegan, who was out with an injury at the time, and got on with getting changed.

The weird thing was that once I'd been told I was in the team it felt as though I'd been there all my life. The most nervous I felt during the whole afternoon was when we went out for the pre-match warm-up, but I really enjoyed the match itself. The thing I remember most about the United team that day was how well Joe Jordan played. We scored our goal with just seven minutes to go, taking the lead through Nicky Holmes, who hit an unstoppable 25-yard shot. Because it was so late in the game we all thought it would be enough to win us the match, but then, with just a couple of minutes to go, a ball fell loose to Joe and he rammed it home. Joe was all-action throughout the game, and although I had no way of knowing it at the time, a few years later I would be the one trying to help him score goals, when he signed for Southampton. There were some other good players in the United side of course, and it was a genuine thrill for me to be on the same pitch with the likes of Steve Coppell, Lou Macari and Sammy McIlroy. Arthur Albiston marked me that day, and he let me know he was there from the start, but I think I gave as good as I got. I was determined that nothing was going to stop me from enjoying myself and making the most of the opportunity Lawrie had given me. The scoreline was a disappointment for us as a team, but nothing could spoil the day for me.

I've always wished I could remember more details about the game, but unfortunately it really did seem to go by in a flash. I've seen a bit of the TV footage a few times, but it was as if I was watching a game of football that didn't really include me. It's still difficult to get my head around the fact that I was a sixteen-year-old kid making my debut at Old Trafford. The whole thing was more in the realm of Roy of the Rovers than reality, but I knew it had happened, and on the way back to the south coast the experience started to catch up with me. I slept like a baby all the way back, then made my way to the digs.

It was a magical day for me, but because mobile phones weren't around then I had to wait until after the match to let my mum and dad know what had happened. They were also able to see me that night on TV. I was interviewed by John Motson for *Match of the Day* after the game, along with Reuben and Lawrie. It was a bit daunting facing the cameras but I enjoyed it, although I did refer to the manager as 'Lawrie' during the interview and got a playful clip round the ear from the big man for my trouble. 'Hey, I'm the boss, and don't forget it!' he said. I suppose I was still on a bit of a high the next day, and of course I looked at all the Sunday papers to see what they said about the game and my performance. The fact that I was so young was a real novelty and it meant that I was mentioned in all of them. They all seemed to think I had done a decent job and hadn't looked out of place in such illustrious company.

I was straight back in for training on the Monday. The rest of the apprentices were really pleased for me. There was no sense of them being jealous, and there was no way I was going to get carried away by what had happened and start getting big-headed. Training again with them brought my feet back down to earth, though it soon became apparent, when I was called in to train with the first team later that week, that I was in line to make a second senior appearance in a week, this time at home against Coventry. It was a funny feeling to be laying out the kit for the first team one day and the next being called in to train with them, but I just got on with it and enjoyed the experience. I never once thought that I'd arrived and was going to be in the side on a regular basis, of course. I was aware that injuries meant this was more of a lucky break for me, and I was just concentrating on not letting myself down. I got a great reception from the Southampton fans when I ran out on to the pitch for the first time at The Dell, which was a taste of things to come for me, because they always treated me well. I think I had a really good relationship with the supporters during the time I was with the club.

That 1–0 win against Coventry on 6 December 1980 ended my brief flirtation with life as a first-team player that season, but it certainly whetted my appetite. I loved every minute of it and knew that if I buckled down and got on with the rest of my time in the youth team I had a good chance of progressing and making it as a full-time professional at the club. I think getting those two games so early in my career also sent out a signal to the rest of the young players, because they could see that if they proved they were good enough, Lawrie McMenemy was the sort of manager who was not afraid to give them their chance. Lawrie never said anything to me about the way I'd played in those two league games, and he never told me that I wouldn't be in the team after the Coventry match, but I knew that as soon as Kevin Keegan was fit again he would be back in the side. I was always a confident player, but that didn't mean I wasn't realistic enough to know that a fit Keegan was always going to be ahead of me in the pecking order.

Getting back to playing in youth-team games was not a problem for me. I enjoyed playing football, and I enjoyed learning about the game from the coaching staff at the club. George Horsfall was the man in charge of the apprentices, and he was terrific with the kids. I think we all learnt a lot from him. Apart from being a good coach who always made training interesting and enjoyable, George also gave us a lot of encouragement, and when you're in your teens trying to gain a secure foothold in the game it's so important to have someone like that who you know is really on your side and wants you to succeed as much as you do. I also got the chance to play in the reserves, which was another valuable experience for me, because quite often the reserves featured experienced players. Whenever I could, I would try to watch the senior players in training too. Fridays were a particular favourite of mine if Southampton were playing a home game the next day. As an apprentice it was my job to go to The Dell anyway and make sure the dressing rooms were in perfect condition for Saturday, but once I'd done my chores I used to like sneaking off to the small gym the first team used for a five-a-side game as part of their training. It was a tiny place, and I would open the door and peek inside, the players often going at it hammer and tongs. It may have been just 24 hours before a big match but there was no holding back. It always seemed incredible to me that there were no serious injuries during those sessions.

Towards the end of that 1980/81 season a familiar face returned to the club: Alan Ball came back after just under a year as Blackpool's player-manager. It was Bally, together with the likes of Kevin Keegan and Mick Channon, who formed the core of Lawrie's side at that time. Not just in the way they played on the pitch, but because they all got on so well with the manager. You could see that he paid a lot of attention to what they said. They were the leaders of the team without any doubt. They had a lot of influence, and from Lawrie's point of view he must have been delighted to have players with their ability and experience around. There were also some good home-grown players coming through, and despite the fact that Southampton were not one of the fashionable clubs and also had limited financial resources, they still managed to finish in sixth place in the league that season – above the likes of Nottingham Forest, Manchester United, Leeds and Spurs – and qualify for Europe. It was a tremendous achievement for the club, and the fact that it had happened under the management of Lawrie McMenemy did not go unnoticed.

CHAPTER FOUR

BIG MAC

After just one season as a Southampton player it was pretty clear to me what an important figure Lawrie McMenemy was at the club. But in the summer of 1981 it suddenly started to look as though the big man would be swapping The Dell for Old Trafford. Manchester United decided to part company with their manager Dave Sexton, and Lawrie was the man they seemed to be targeting to replace him. It wasn't just rumour either. But, even though it must have been a tough decision for him to make, Lawrie eventually turned down the chance to move north and manage one of the biggest clubs in the world in favour of sticking with what he knew at Southampton.

I don't know how it would have affected my career had he gone, but considering how things went for me in the years that followed, I can only be pleased and grateful that he decided to stay. Lawrie had shown enough faith to push me into the first team for those two games the previous season, so I knew I had a chance of making the grade under him if I continued to learn my trade at the club. Another manager might have had different ideas and not have fancied me, so it could all have been very different. I do know that everyone at the club seemed to be happy that Lawrie decided to stay. He'd become Mr Southampton since taking over in 1973, and because of his regular appearances on TV as a football expert he was also probably one of the sport's best-known faces and personalities. It all added to his aura at The Dell as far as the youngsters were concerned, and there was never any question about who ran the club. As I got to know him better over the years I realised that you could hardly call him a tracksuit manager. I don't think his strength was coaching, but he was a very good tactician and second to none when it came to man-management. In many ways he was very much like someone else who I was to play for later in my career, Sir Alex Ferguson, who is also a formidable man-manager and who knew exactly how to set up his teams. Lawrie was not the sort of person you would see a lot of on the training ground during the week – he would leave that to his coach, Lew Chatterley – but he dictated tactics and decided on the shape and set-up of the side.

My life as a second-season apprentice started less spectacularly, but I knew I was doing well and once again I managed to get a few games in the reserves as well. My big chance came towards the end of that 1981/82 season, when I was picked for the away match with Notts County on 6 March. Although I was substituted in the 1–1 draw, I managed to do enough to retain my place for the next match, against Sunderland four days later, which we lost 2–0. I think Lawrie just wanted to have a look at me again to see how I coped with the big-match atmosphere and a better standard of player, and I went out on both occasions determined to make sure I stayed in his memory. After those two games I stayed on the fringes of things for the rest of the season, making only one more start in the first team and figuring as a substitute on four other occasions. I wouldn't say I'd arrived, but I did feel I was in there with a good chance when the 1982/83 season began.

Backing up that belief was the fact that I had been given my first full-time professional contract as a nice New Year's present. I was only just eighteen. After starting off being paid £28 a week I'd been given a wage rise of £7 a week at the start of my second year with the club. But when I was told in January 1982 that I was going to be earning £75 a week, I could hardly believe it. The money seemed like a fortune, and considering my age and the fact that I was still living in digs, I felt as if I'd hit the jackpot. When you live in digs, as I said, the club pay for all the meals provided for you, which means the only money you really spend goes on things like clothes and going out with your mates. The wage increase, coupled with the fact that I'd made it into the first team again in the spring, meant that I felt pretty good about things as the close season approached. Indeed, when the new campaign started a couple of months later, I soon realised that things were suddenly starting to happen for me.

It was during that summer of 1982 that two of the biggest names in the club departed. Mick Channon had been brilliant for the club since returning from Manchester City, so I think it surprised quite a few people when he went. But the move that really caused a stir was Kevin Keegan leaving. He played a few pre-season games and then went to Newcastle. The news upset a lot of Southampton fans who had already bought season tickets thinking they would again be seeing him in action, but it probably wasn't as surprising inside the club, because Keegan and Lawrie had not seen eye to eye for a few months following a home game with Aston Villa in April.

As I've already said, Southampton had a pretty good team at the time with a real mixture of youth and experience, and for that game I was part of the youth of the team. That Villa game was my third start of the season, so it was all still very much a new experience for me. The match was at The Dell, and we went into it in third place in Division One with people expecting the team to do well, but the game was disastrous for us and we lost 3–0. Lawrie had a real go at everyone in the dressing room afterwards. He didn't actually have a go at anyone individually, claiming instead that we were all useless and hadn't tried hard enough. It was the first time I'd seen him tear into people like that, and when you're only eighteen it's all a bit overwhelming, I can tell you. I just sat quietly and kept my head down, not wanting to attract any attention to myself. I knew I had tried my hardest out there on the pitch and given everything I'd got, but I wasn't about to start arguing with the manager. But that wasn't the case with Kevin Keegan, who was experienced and confident enough not to let Lawrie's remarks pass. He was also pretty stubborn when he had an opinion. He got upset at Lawrie's suggestion that he hadn't tried because that was something he always did. When Keegan played he gave everything, so he took exception to the fact that someone was questioning his commitment in that way. Pretty much from that moment on there was silence between the two men; I don't think either of them spoke to each other for quite some time.

Still, for me, getting the chance to play alongside Kevin Keegan was a huge thrill. One of the games I remember most during his time with the club was a midweek match at home with Coventry, near the end of Keegan's stay at The Dell. After the 90 minutes was up the scoreline stood at 5–5. The goals had been flying in so thick and fast, and I'd been so wrapped up in the action, that when the final whistle was blown I wasn't at all sure of the exact score. After the game Lawrie came into the dressing room and was really upset that we hadn't gone on and won the match instead of drawing. Now, I've always been quiet in the dressing room, but on this occasion I couldn't help blurting out from my seat in the corner, 'Drawing? I thought we lost!' The whole dressing room erupted with laughter.

Lawrie's experience with Keegan certainly didn't put him off signing well-established, high-profile internationals: he went out and brought England keeper Peter Shilton to the club, and he also drafted in Justin Fashanu on loan from Nottingham Forest. We had a lot to look forward to as the new season started because Southampton were also in Europe and had been drawn against the Swedish part-timers IFK Norrkoping in the first round of the UEFA Cup. The good thing from my point of view was that despite the poor team performance against Villa in the last full game I'd played, the manager still seemed to like what he saw and kept me around things when it came to the first team. I didn't start any games early in that 1982/83 season, but you can just imagine how pleased I was to be included in the squad for the legs against Norrkoping on 15 and 29 September. Any player will tell you that playing in European competitions is a bit special, and when you're as young as I was the thought of being involved in something like that was incredibly exciting.

I'd actually got my first real taste of European football the season before, when I came on as a late substitute in our second-round second-leg UEFA Cup game against Sporting Lisbon in Portugal. We'd lost the first match 4–2 at The Dell, and could only manage a goalless draw in the return, which meant we got knocked out. But the worst thing was that I got absolutely slaughtered by Lawrie after the game. Obviously I was young and inexperienced, but he was really unhappy with the fact that I'd sauntered over for a corner late in the game and taken so much time when we were desperate for goals. The game was played in front of 60,000 people – a really big occasion. Norrkoping were hardly in the same league as Sporting Lisbon, and I wanted to make up for what had happened during my brief appearance in the competition the previous season. It should have been an experience that stayed in my mind for all the right reasons, but unfortunately it turned out to provide one of the scariest moments of my young life, and it ended with me thinking that I might have blown any chance I ever had of making it with Southampton.

The first thing to go wrong was the result of the first leg, a game in which I didn't play. We could only manage a 2–2 draw against this team of part-timers, but footballers being footballers, we certainly didn't let that get the better of us. After all, there was still the trip to Sweden to come a fortnight later, and we weren't going to miss out on sampling some of the delights of Swedish nightlife. Sure enough, after that second leg was over we all went out and had a good time. I was just happy to tag along and have a few drinks and a laugh. I was pleased to be involved; there was never any sense that I was excluded from anything. There was a team mentality about everything we did, on and off the pitch.

We got back to the hotel in good spirits, Swedish hospitality having helped us to cheer up after a dismal 0–0 draw that allowed Norrkoping to progress in the competition on the away-goals rule. I went back to my room and got into bed, but I could hear noises coming from along the corridor, some shouting and yelling. I went to investigate and soon found that our striker, Steve Moran, had a girl in his room. It may not sound very gentlemanly, but once we found out what was going on it seemed to be the signal for a few of us to go along to his room to have a look at what was happening. Not all the players piled in to have a look, and perhaps if I'd been a bit older and wiser I wouldn't have got involved, but I was a kid who just wanted to be part of everything, however stupid and wrong that may seem. There was lots of shouting and jokes from the players who had gone to the room. It wasn't particularly clever, but things like that have gone on over the years with groups of blokes, especially if they are in football or rugby teams. It was dirty schoolboy stuff, boys behaving badly, something I should have steered clear of but didn't.

What had seemed like a bit of fun the night before turned into a nightmare the next morning when Steve and defender Mark Wright were arrested by the local police on a sexual assault charge. It must have been particularly frightening for Mark because he wasn't even in the room at the time! Along with the accusation, the girl in Steve's bed had also told the police that several of his team-mates were involved as well. In her statement she mentioned two black players, and as Reuben Agboola and I were the only two black lads in the squad it was pretty clear who she was referring to. The police detained Steve and Mark and we had to fly home without them. When we got to the airport I was convinced I was going to be arrested. I knew I hadn't done anything wrong, other than look on as part of a rowdy group of blokes who thought it was all a bit of a laugh, but that didn't stop me being scared stiff.

As things turned out I wasn't arrested, but that didn't mean I was off the hook as far as Lawrie McMenemy was concerned. The fact that we'd also been dumped out of the UEFA Cup at the first hurdle didn't help to lift his black mood. When I got back to Southampton he went berserk, and fined me for what had gone on. He knew I'd been stupid and was livid with the fact that I'd allowed myself to get involved in something like that. Alan Ball said I was naive and he hoped I'd learnt a lesson, but he was really good to me and told me not to worry. Still, I honestly thought that was going to be the end of my Southampton career. Steve and Mark were later cleared of the assault charge, but the episode showed just how easily a bunch of footballers can get themselves into trouble.

To be fair to Lawrie, once he had dealt with the situation and made sure I knew just how stupid I had been, he kept me in and around the first team and allowed my career to flourish. On 23 October I started the match away at Swansea. We lost 3–2, but from a personal point of view it was really a turning point in my career. I thought the goal I got against Swansea, my first in the league, was going to earn us a point, but they scored with just two minutes to go to grab a win. Justin Fashanu, in what was to be his last game for the club, scored our first goal, hooking the ball home from eighteen yards out, but then the Welsh side scored twice through an own-goal by Dennis Rofe and a strike by Leighton James. Seven minutes after the break came my big moment. A long through-ball was cleared out of defence and I ran on to it. In a split second I could feel one of their defenders trying to get a tackle in on me, but he couldn't quite reach me, and as the keeper came off his line to try to smother my shot I just placed it past him and into the net. It was a fantastic feeling, and we all thought we were going to hang on for a draw, until Jimmy Loveridge popped up with the winner for them late on. In our next outing a week later I got another, when we beat Everton by the same score at The Dell. From that point on I never really looked back. For the rest of the season I was a regular fixture in the team, and I finished with 32 league games under my belt, as well as twelve goals, which made me Southampton's top scorer in the league. By the time my nineteenth birthday came round in January 1983 I was earning good money, playing regularly in the First Division, and the media were talking about me as a real prospect.

Although it was all going well for me, I wasn't the sort of person to get carried away by sudden fame. That doesn't mean I didn't enjoy it, of course, but I didn't go out and get a flashy car or house. In fact, I couldn't even drive at the time. I think I might have caused a few raised eyebrows once I'd got into the first team on a regular basis because I still used to turn up and go home from matches on a bus. I'm sure a few fans might have done a double-take and wondered what I was doing, but I never gave it a second thought. I'd always used public transport; it was second nature to me to hop on a bus if I wanted to get around Southampton. And fans' attention was another new aspect of me being a first-team player that I had to get used to, particularly female fans. I would certainly never claim to be the best-looking guy in the world, but it didn't seem to matter too much what I looked like; the simple fact that I was a footballer meant

I got a lot more attention than I would have done had I had a less high-profile job. Certain girls liked to be seen with footballers, and as a healthy young man I wasn't about to turn my back on all the attention that suddenly started to come my way.

Despite the fact that I was living in Southampton and Jenny was still in London, we managed to maintain our relationship, although I suppose there was a kind of agreement that we would see other people if we wanted to. We were both very young, and I'm sure if that hadn't been the case our relationship would have gone out of the window pretty quickly. I continued to go up to London to see Jenny, and there was never really any talk about us breaking up. We carried on the long-distance relationship just as we had from the very first day I signed for the club. Having said that, as my local fame grew it did start to change things for us, as we would discover over the coming months.

As the new 1983/84 season approached I was offered a new contract by the club. My £75 per week still seemed like a good wage to me, but the new deal helped me to feel as though I'd won the jackpot: I was going to get £200 per week, which was great money. What Lawrie McMenemy and the club didn't realise was that the extra cash would be particularly useful, because that June Jenny and I became the proud parents of a baby boy who we called Remi. Jen and I might have had a long-distance relationship, but it hadn't stopped us facing the prospect of being a mum and dad.

As crazy as it may seem, nothing much changed. I continued to live in my Southampton digs, and Jenny got a flat in New Cross for her and the baby. It seems incredible to me now that I could have been so self-centred. I was focused on my career, and on continuing the lifestyle I had; I might have just become a father, but as far as I was concerned the whole thing was at arm's length. And, despite having to bring Remi up on her own to begin with, Jenny wasn't unhappy with the arrangement. She was a South London girl, and the thought of moving down to somewhere like Southampton wasn't that appealing to her. I also think she liked her independence. She has always been very strong-minded and determined. If she had not been happy with the arrangement Jenny would certainly have let me know. She had her own life and a job in London, as well as her own group of friends. Jenny was also heavily into acting, and was part of the Drama and Dance group that performed regularly at the Albany Empire in Deptford. She had real talent, and some of her friends in the group went on to become professional actors: Kim Walker was in the comedy series *Desmond's*, Eamonn Walker acted in *The Bill*, and Frank Harper was in the film *Lock, Stock and Two Smoking Barrels*. I think Jenny would have loved to have a career as an actress. She played the part of a pregnant junkie in one of the Albany Empire productions while she was carrying Remi, and after a successful audition she got the chance to tour with a play, but it was just at the time when he was born. It would have led to her getting her Equity card, but she had to pass up the opportunity because of the responsibility of looking after the baby. It didn't really mean much to me then, but I have since thought about the fact that even at that stage in her life Jenny was making sacrifices for me and her children.

To be honest, it's amazing that we managed to stay together. But perhaps it was all meant to be, and I'm glad for it. Jenny means the world to me, and without her help and love I dread to think what might have happened to me in recent years. There must have been plenty of times during our relationship when it could all have gone wrong, and I know I've given her more than enough cause during our time together to walk out on me and not come back. I'm so lucky that we've stayed together. My only regret is that I didn't have the maturity in those early days to treat her better. It wasn't that I didn't love her, it was more a case of me wanting the best of both worlds. I was happy enough to have a baby, but I also wanted the lifestyle of a single young man to go with it. Having Jenny and Remi in London while I was in Southampton seemed like the perfect arrangement. The fact that I had the money to support Jenny probably helped, but looking back there was no excuse for not setting up home together as soon as the baby arrived.

Both Jenny's parents and my own were pleased and proud to be grandparents – or at least they were by the time of the birth. Jenny was still living at home with her mum and dad around the time of conception. Several weeks later she had a feeling that she might be pregnant, so she went to the doctor to have a test, but in those days it took a week before the results came through. Jenny's mum didn't need that long to recognise her daughter's condition. She'd had twelve kids of her own so I suppose she knew a thing or two about pregnancy, and she was obviously spot on. I don't think she was that happy to begin with, mostly because of the fact that we were so young, but there was never any question of an abortion, and once they had got over the shock her parents were really supportive.

My poor mum was very upset when she found out, but that was because of the way she got to know about the pregnancy. It wasn't that she didn't want us to have a baby, it was simply that I hadn't told her about it. She found out when one of my cousins saw Jen in the high street when she was about seven months gone and put two and two together. It was another case of me being stupid and not thinking properly. I suppose I was a bit concerned about what my parents' reaction might be when they found out, so I didn't tell them. It just goes to show how young and immature I was. I was in Southampton for most of the time so it was easy for me to bury my head in the sand instead of facing up to what was about to happen and take some responsibility. I didn't actually get to the hospital to see Remi being born, but the next day I travelled up to London and met my mum before going along to see Jenny and the baby. I was thrilled when I saw Remi, and I could see Mum was happy and proud as well. All the unhappiness of not knowing about the pregnancy for so long had disappeared by this time and it was obvious she was really pleased, even if the child's mum and dad weren't going to be living together.

So, back in Southampton I continued my single ways, although Jenny did start to visit me on some weekends. We both enjoyed going out to clubs and having a drink, so whenever we could get a baby-sitter for Remi we took the opportunity to hit the town and visit some of the nightspots. It might not have been what Jenny was used to in London, but she soon began to enjoy Southampton, despite there being the complication of other girls floating around.

They obviously didn't realise I had a regular girlfriend and would come up and start talking to me even though Jenny was right beside me. It didn't take Jen long to put a few of them in their place. If they were silly enough to answer back she wasn't averse to physically emphasising the point she was trying to make. I saw her dish out a slap on more than one occasion just to make sure they realised I was spoken for.

Of course, it didn't stop me getting friendly with the local girls once Jenny was back in London. I just looked on it as harmless fun and thought I was being smart – until Jenny caught me out. I had met a girl in Southampton and gone out with her on a few occasions, and one day about six months after Remi was born Jenny found her number on a piece of paper which fell out of my jacket pocket. She decided to do her own bit of detective work, dialled the number and heard a female voice answer the phone. She told me later that she instinctively knew it was someone I had been seeing behind her back, and that she'd let the girl know in no uncertain terms what she had let herself in for. 'If you really want him you can have him,' she told her. 'But perhaps you'd also like to know that he has a six-month-old baby as well.' The double barrelled verbal blast and the information that I was also a father was enough to frighten the girl off and things ended there and then. Perhaps things like that would have been enough to end the relationship for other couples, but Jenny and I carried on. I think the fact that there was literally so much space between us geographically was a major factor. There always seemed to be a freshness whenever we met up.

Because Remi arrived in the close season it was easier for me to keep his birth quiet. Hard as it may be to believe, nobody at the club, including Lawrie McMenemy, knew that their bright young goalscoring wing prospect had become a dad. I've already mentioned how Lawrie seemed to be Mr Southampton, and you could see the way he'd stamped his character on pretty much everything that went on at the club. Although he'd never actually said anything to me directly about families and children, I think I knew his feelings on the importance of a family and the responsibilities that went with having kids. Maybe that was why I never said anything to him about Remi. Perhaps in the back of my mind I was a bit scared about his reaction to what had happened and the fact that I had no intention of bringing Jenny down to live with me. If I'm honest, I was being selfish again. I didn't want anything to rock the boat. Telling Lawrie about the baby might have complicated things, and I just wanted to concentrate on my football.

When I turned up for pre-season training about a month after the birth I chatted about everything and anything with the rest of the players as we caught up with what had been going on in our lives during the summer, but I didn't tell anyone about the fact that I now had a son. I shake my head when I think about it now, but believe it or not, it didn't seem a strange thing to do at the time. My life was all about football, and having had such a good season in 1982/83 and established myself in the first team, I was determined to prove that I was no one-season wonder. I was nineteen years old, and I felt that the footballing world was literally at my feet. I'd had a taste of what it was like to play regularly in the English First Division and I'd proved that I could handle myself against the best players in the country. Lawrie had had enough faith in me to give me my chance as a regular first-team player once Alan Ball had left the club to play in Hong Kong, and I hadn't disappointed him. I'd ended the campaign with twelve goals and I couldn't wait to get started again.

CHAPTER FIVE

DELL BOYS

The team I'd been a part of in 1982/83 was a pretty good one, but we'd finished in mid-table and during the summer it was clear that Lawrie was keen to try and put together a side that would do a lot better the next time out. There was a bit of a change-around on the playing and coaching staff, with the likes of Chris Nicholl, who had been our regular centre-half, moving to Grimsby and Lawrie bringing in a real character in the shape of veteran striker Frank Worthington. Having someone like him around was not only great on the playing side of things, it was also good off the field because of his extrovert personality. Once again it showed Lawrie's ability to blend experience with youth and also to get the best out of big-name players. Peter Shilton had done brilliantly, not only on the pitch but also in terms of his presence off it, since coming to the club the year before; England defender Mick Mills was another player who had joined the previous season and had a positive effect. But we also had some good young players like Steve Moran, Steve Williams and Mark Wright. It was a good blend, and one which was to go on and produce one of the best seasons in the club's history.

Having players like Shilton and Worthington around was great for someone like me. Shilts was incredible in the way he went about his job. Everyone knew what a great keeper he was, but it wasn't until you trained and played with him on a regular basis that you realised how professional he was in terms of his approach. He liked to leave nothing to chance and worked really hard on the training pitch. He also had his own set way of preparing on a match day, and nothing ever seemed to interrupt his routine. I think he knew he was naturally a great keeper, but it didn't stop him working each and every day to make sure he maintained the level of consistency that had brought him so much success. As far as he was concerned, he was always prepared and would do his job for the team; it was then up to the rest of the team to make sure they did their job as well.

Frank Worthington came across as a very laid-back person, but he loved the game and he also gave everything when he was on the pitch. He was one of the most skilful players I've ever seen. Even though his best days were behind him when he arrived at The Dell, there was no mistaking his class, or his charisma. Frank was full of neat little tricks and flicks on the pitch and he could pass the ball very well. He had a reputation as a bit of a playboy and showman, and although he often lived up to those labels, it didn't stop him being devoted to football and being as competitive as anyone else on the field. We used to call him Elvis, because whenever he could Frank would be blasting out Presley's music. I think he loved Elvis Presley as much as he loved football and having a good time off the park. He was a real character, and would turn up for games wearing his little shoelace neck-ties. I think he would have loved to be a rock and roll star, and if he had been as good with a guitar and a microphone as he was with a football I've no doubt the lifestyle would have suited him down to the ground. Frank was perfect for us at that time, and his flair certainly gave the team an added dimension. David Armstrong, who was a good striker, certainly benefited from his arrival. Having someone with Frank's experience and cunning on the pitch really helped turn us from being a decent side into a good one.

Lawrie also brought in defender Ken Armstrong from Kilmarnock for about £50,000. He did a really good job for us at the back along with either Mark Wright or Reuben Agboola, and in November 1983 another character hit the south coast, Mark Dennis. Although Stuart Pearce later picked up the nickname 'Psycho' for the way he played, it was Mark who got the original 'Psycho' tag. He arrived at Southampton from Birmingham with a reputation as a fierce-tackling left-back who had disciplinary problems, but once again Lawrie showed he wasn't afraid to take a gamble, and also that he wasn't worried by reputations. He got the best out of Mark during the time he was in charge of him, and although most of the headlines Dennis got seemed to be for his tackling or for discipline, I can tell you that he was one of the most skilful full-backs I've ever come across. In fact, for a couple of years I'm convinced there wasn't a better full-back in the country. I used to feel sorry for him in many ways, because all people wanted to talk about when they discussed him was the way he could cut a winger in half with one of his challenges. What so many people seemed to miss or gloss over was the fact that he could really play, and his style suited the team perfectly at that time. Mark was an honest, down-to-earth guy. He loved his football and he enjoyed relaxing off the pitch with a few drinks. Like me, he was a South London boy, and we got on well together, although I have to admit I preferred playing on his side rather than having to face him, as I sometimes did during training. There was no doubt that, in the best possible way, Mark was a bit crazy.

I remember he once went into a tackle in his normal fashion, and although he won the ball, he came off second best physically because he had to be substituted after getting a dead leg. As if that wasn't bad enough, the leg soon started to swell, and it was clear he would have to go to hospital to have it drained. It wasn't the sort of way Mark wanted to spend a Saturday night, and when his wife, Jane, arrived at the hospital, Psycho was propped up in a bed with his leg bandaged and was expected to have to stay in overnight until the swelling subsided enough for him to go home. But that thought didn't appeal to Mark, so with the aid of a wheelchair he left the hospital and spent the rest of the night drinking in a local pub with Jane!

There was another player who was just beginning to build a reputation for himself at the club that season when he was signed as an apprentice. His name was Dennis Wise, and you could see there was no holding him back. He was about as small as me, but it soon became clear he was the top dog among the rest of the new intake. I think he even had a run-in or two with Lawrie McMenemy during the couple of years he was with the club, before moving on to Wimbledon and then Chelsea. Also in the junior ranks that season were my twin brothers Rodney and Raymond, who in December followed in my footsteps and signed associate schoolboy forms with Southampton. They had taken pretty much the same route as me, with Rod showing real ability as a striker and Ray going against the trend a bit by playing as a defender or midfielder. Having three brothers at the same club was a bit of a novelty, and I'm sure Mum and Dad were proud of all three of their Dell boys.

I really enjoyed that second season in the first team, especially as we did so well in the league. One game that really stood out for me was the 8–2 home victory over Coventry City in late April. It was one of those games where everything I tried seemed to come off. I scored three goals and made all the others, including providing the passes for Steve Moran to score a hat-trick. Dave Armstrong and Frank Worthington got the other goals, and I was absolutely delighted when the final whistle went and we'd managed such a fantastic win. It is, of course, tradition for someone who scores a hat-trick to get the match ball signed by all the players, but when I looked around for it at the end of the game I saw Steve wandering off with it under his arm. I didn't want to make a fuss, but I have to admit that I was disappointed. Steve seemed determined to keep it, but in the dressing room Dave said that he should give it to me because the hat-trick I'd scored was my first for the club. Suddenly, the rest of the lads started to agree with him. In the end Steve had to hand the ball over to me, but I don't think he was happy! It turned out to be my first and last hat-trick for the club in the league, although I did score two others in Cup matches – against Middlesborough in the FA Cup and Stoke in the Full Members' Cup. And in that Coventry match it was also the first time in almost two decades that two Southampton forwards had scored hat-tricks for the club in the same game.

It was no fluke that we finished the season just three points behind Liverpool, who won the championship. It was the club's best ever campaign in the league and there was quite a bit of celebrating in the dressing room following the final game of the season at Notts County, after we had beaten them 3–1. I was really disappointed in April when Everton beat us in our FA Cup semi-final – the only goal of the game, scored by Adrian Heath, came during extra-time –

because ever since I was a kid it had been my dream to play in an FA Cup final at Wembley. I'd always watched the match on TV and had always imagined myself one day scoring the winner and walking up those famous steps to collect the cup and my winner's medal. But I just had to accept it wasn't to be that year.

Personally, I had a really good season. I missed only one game in the league and netted eleven goals in the process, which made me third top scorer for Southampton behind Dave Armstrong and Steve Moran. Once again I'd really enjoyed myself in the First Division and had proved that I was not out of place with some of the seasoned players around. And things are harder in the second year. A good new player who has just come on to the scene has a decent chance of getting the best out of a situation, but second time round defenders in particular are much more aware of the threat you pose. In my case that would often mean teams trying to double up on me, making sure that if I got past one defender there was another player ready to challenge me. That never really bothered me, though: I used to love pitting myself against a full-back and trying to get one over on him during a game. The fact that I was pretty small never bothered me either. I was always a competitor and I was never afraid to get stuck in and tackle people, although I could never claim to be the world's best when it came to tracking back and defending. Obviously some players were better at stopping me than others, but I always felt I gave as good as I got, even against the best of them.

My second season was also the first time I came across Stuart Pearce, who had joined Coventry after playing non-league football. I can honestly say that he was one of the few players who frightened me. When he came in for a tackle you knew that he was going to go right through you. He wasn't dirty, he was just determined to get the ball at all costs, and most of the time that meant he got the ball, plus you and anything else that stood in his way. When he hit you, there was no doubt in your mind that you had been tackled. It could literally take your breath away. But if I did get splattered I always got back up and got on with it. There's nothing more disheartening for a full-back than to see a winger taking him on all the time and not being put off by any of the tackles he's dishing out.

Another player who was a hard tackler was Everton's John Bailey. He was a very solid player, and although I would always fancy my chances against him, I knew that if he did catch me I'd know all about it. He played against us in the cup semi-final at Highbury and I think we both knew we'd been in a game at the end of it. Viv Anderson was another defender I always had a battle with. Viv was a tall, gangly player, and not only was he a quick and hard tackler, he also had the ability to drag one of those long legs of his out and catch you just when you thought you had the ball.

I had respect for players like Bailey, Pearce, Anderson and the rest of the full-backs in the First Division, but it didn't stop me thinking I was going to get the better of them every time I went out on to the football field. I wasn't cocky, but I was certainly confident, and the fact that I was still only twenty years old and playing against some very good defenders didn't mean that much to me. I never stopped to think about what had happened since I joined Southampton, or how quickly. I didn't really feel any different playing a match at Highbury or Old Trafford to the way I'd felt running about the pitch as a school kid. It all just seemed so natural to me, and I think I took everything in my stride. I was just having fun and playing the game I'd always loved. Life couldn't have been better for me. I didn't have a care in the world. But I was about to get a reality check and a lesson in how being a professional footballer isn't all about just playing football.

The fact that there was still nobody at the club who knew I had a baby was amazing considering all the gossiping that goes on and the daily banter that takes place in any football dressing room. I certainly hadn't let anyone know about it, and whenever Jenny came to visit me in Southampton, Remi usually stayed in London with her family, which meant that when anyone saw us out and about we looked like any other young couple on a date. And, as I said, I was still living the life of a single man without any ties. I loved Jen and I loved the baby, but when I was in Southampton on my own I'm afraid to say that didn't stop me behaving like a complete idiot on occasions. I met girls and continued to see them, even though Jenny and Remi were back in London and I now had responsibilities. It was a situation that was always likely to end in tears.

One day a national newspaper took a picture of Jenny in a park with Remi and were going to run a story about me having a kid. The reason the paper had the story was because they had been tipped off by one of the girls I had been seeing, and she had found out about the baby. I think the paper were going to run a 'love rat' type piece, saying that I had a girlfriend and baby in London yet I was still carrying on with different girls in Southampton. It's a situation that would have meant little had I been an electrician or a mechanic, but I was a professional footballer playing in the First Division, and that was something a paper could make a big thing out of.

To this day I don't know how or why, but Lawrie McMenemy managed to get wind of the fact that there was trouble brewing and something was about to be printed. He hauled me into his office and told me exactly what I was going to do. I was going to send for Jenny and the baby, the club were going to rent a house for us, and the three of us were going to start living together as a family. I could see that it wasn't just a case of Lawrie acting the boss and laying down the law to one of his young players. It was more than that. He was genuinely a great believer in family values. In many ways I think that was why Southampton had the feel of a family club about it. As I've said, he gave the place its direction and set the tone. He clearly didn't like the thought of Jenny and me being so far away from each other when we had a kid to bring up, and I think he also wanted to make sure that I realised I couldn't distance myself from the whole thing. I had responsibilities, and I had to face up to them. It wasn't just about Jenny, Remi and me, it was about me growing up and maturing as a man, and I think he believed that having the two of them living with me would speed up that process. He wanted to see Jenny as well, just to let her know about his proposal and what the club were going to do. You could tell he was concerned for her. I'm sure he thought she shouldn't have to put up with having her private life splashed across a tabloid newspaper. I'm not sure exactly what happened, but the story never appeared. Lawrie certainly saw the pictures they had taken of the three of us because he had them on his desk when he spoke to Jenny and me. I don't know whether he was able to have a word with someone and persuade them not to take the story any further, but I do know it was the last we heard of it, and pretty soon we were moving into new accommodation in Romsey.

I'm sure it was a bit of a shock to the system for Jenny. She was a South London girl and she loved living there. She had the support of her family who were just a few minutes away from where she lived, and she felt secure. Although she had visited Southampton a lot, it was only for a couple of days at a time; actually living in the place was a different proposition. It wasn't such a problem for me, of course. I had the advantage of having lived in the city for several years, and of being able to concentrate on my football. I got up in the morning and went to training, leaving Jenny and the baby behind. That's almost certainly something a lot of footballers' wives have to deal with, especially when a player moves to a new area after being transferred, but at the time we just got on with it and Jenny began to deal with a completely new way of life.

In the afternoons, Jenny, Remi and I went for walks and looked at different houses to buy. We appreciated the fact that the club had set us up in a rented place, but we both wanted our own home and I was earning enough money for us to be able to look at some decent places in the area. I started to enjoy family life, even though it wasn't quite as ordinary and settled as it might sound. Jen and I were both twenty years old and neither of us was that mature, but we were in the middle of a world where I could make news by getting a ticket for speeding. Playing football for a living was all I'd ever wanted to do, but coming to terms with some of the things that went with that wasn't always easy. Southampton isn't a big place, and because it only has one football team the players are easily recognised in the area. That can be great sometimes, but it also means that your privacy is restricted and doing normal things like eating in restaurants, having a drink in a pub or going to a club can be problematic.

Happily, Jenny soon made friends with some of the other players' wives and girlfriends through going to watch home games, but she has always been the sort of person who has kept to her own group of long-term friends, girls she has known since she was a kid. And although she used to go to The Dell, Jenny has never been interested in football. She always wanted us to win, and for me to play well without getting injured, but that was about it. The actual game has never excited her, and she's always been the first to admit that. One of the things she enjoyed most about visiting The Dell on match day was the social side of things after the game had finished and everyone was in the bar having a drink. Quite often after that we'd kiss and say goodbye, and Jenny would take Remi and head back to London to have a night out with the girls while I clicked again into single-man mode and went to some clubs in Southampton. A lot of the time I had my mates from London down for the weekend, and they loved having a boys' night out.

It's strange to think how much things have changed during the past twenty years. Of course Premiership footballers still go out after a game, but they pay a lot more attention to what they eat and drink than we did. I certainly wasn't a heavy drinker, but I could booze with the best of them after a match and think nothing of it. Most players would have a few pints after a game and then maybe go out for some more to a bar or club before rounding the night off with a curry. These days it's all about sports drinks and refuelling after a match. Players, managers and coaches are all much more aware of fitness issues and what needs to be done in order to maintain a high level of performance on the pitch. The stakes were always high, but with the introduction of the Premiership and the money involved these days everything has been raised to a new level, and that includes the way players look after themselves. Still, things might have been different for me as a young player, I might have been more likely to have a beer in my hand after a match than a Lucozade, but it didn't seem to affect my performances on the pitch. I had broken into the England set-up at youth level and as an under-21, scoring on my debut at, of all places, Portsmouth's Fratton Park against Greece.

In fact I played regularly for the under-21 side in 1983/84, and some people had even started to suggest that in 1984/85 I might start pushing myself forward for a full cap if I kept up the sort of progress I had made.

There was a new face at the training ground for the start of the new season: Joe Jordan arrived from Verona to replace Frank Worthington, who left the club for Brighton. Although Joe took over from Frank, their styles were very different. Joe was much more aggressive as a player and was one of the bravest strikers I've ever seen. He would put his head to anything and was always prepared to give his all during a game. Defenders hated playing against him because he would never give them a moment's rest. He also looked fearsome on the pitch because he used to take his false front teeth out just before a match. When he came roaring towards the ball for a header he looked like Dracula waiting to pounce rather than a centre-forward trying to score a goal. Joe certainly added a new dimension to our play, and off the pitch we soon learnt that he was a really nice guy who was very knowledgeable about the game. He loved to win and was a real competitor – a characteristic that applied just as much on the training pitch as it did during matches.

I remember being totally shocked one day when we were at the training ground taking part in a five-a-side match. As usual the game was being played at a high tempo with nobody pulling out of tackles. I'm not sure exactly what happened, but suddenly everyone realised there was a commotion going on at one end of the pitch. We all turned round to see George Lawrence, who had come up through the club's youth ranks with me, and Joe Jordan punching lumps out of each other. Our first reaction was to run over and try to break up the fight, but it was as if we all realised at the same moment that because they were big guys we might catch a whack for our troubles. So we all took a step back and waited for them to calm down and the whole thing to fizzle out before carrying on as if nothing had happened. You often get flare-ups in training, but that was the first time I'd experienced it, and I have to admit that I was shocked by the sight of two team-mates fighting on the training pitch.

But if that came as a bit of a shock, it was nothing compared to the time when Mark Wright and Lawrie McMenemy had a punch-up at half-time during a game at The Dell. It happened soon after we'd trooped off the pitch and reached the dressing room. When we got there everyone sat down expecting the usual team talk from Lawrie, but it didn't happen. Instead we could hear the sound of raised voices coming from the area that housed the showers and bath. It wasn't clear what was going on at first or who was shouting at who, but when I got up to have a look my eyes nearly popped out of my head. Wrighty was in there with Lawrie, and they weren't just shouting at each other. Things had got physical, and blows were being exchanged. As we all looked on open-mouthed at what was happening, Mark suddenly grabbed the boss and started to wrestle him, somehow managing to flip Lawrie into the bath, which was full of water. The sight of big Lawrie dragging himself out of the water, dripping wet, is something I will never forget, but none of us had too much time to dwell on these shocking events because we had to go out for the second half. We ran out as if nothing had happened, leaving poor Lawrie to dry himself and find a new set of clothes. I don't remember anything else being said about the incident, and to his credit Lawrie didn't haul Mark off. He stayed on the pitch and played the rest of the game without any of the crowd being aware of what had gone on in the changing room. I don't even know if Mark was disciplined for what he did, or if Lawrie took any other sort of action. Of course I'd seen players having disagreements with him, but that was the first time I'd ever seen anyone raise his hands. And it was certainly the first time Lawrie had ever been thrown in the bath by a player.

I think the way we played that season when Joe Jordan joined us changed in many ways. Frank Worthington was the sort of striker who liked to drop back and thread balls through to other players, in much the same way as Teddy Sheringham has done over the years. He could get on the end of balls as well, but he presented problems for defenders because he wasn't always in their faces and they often had difficulty deciding exactly how to mark him. Frank would make goals for others as well as score them, and he set up so many great moves for us during the course of games. Joe was much more of a traditional centre-forward, albeit a very good one indeed. He was incredibly brave and really led the line. I lost count of the number of times he managed to win the ball when you thought it was a lost cause, and he was always available during a game. He'd do so much unselfish running, and he was brilliant in the air. Because of the way he played, though, I think the team had to change in order to make the most of the qualities he brought with him. But that didn't mean we weren't still a good side. It was always going to be hard to follow what we had done in 1983/84, when we finished second, but by May 1985 we'd secured fifth place in the league having maintained a high level of performance, and we got into Europe again.

What none of us could have known as we went into that season in the summer of 1984 was that it would turn out to be Lawrie's last in charge of the club. After becoming a Southampton legend during twelve years in charge, the big man finally decided that he'd had enough and wanted a new challenge. It came in the form of a chance to sample life as a manager in his native north-east, with Sunderland. And it left Southampton struggling to come to terms with the end of an era.

CHAPTER SIX

BROTHERS IN ARMS

From the very day I signed for Southampton, things had gone well for me. I'd been fortunate to see my first-team career take off at such a young age, and there hadn't been any real set-backs for me to have to cope with. A footballer's life can often be full of ups and downs because there are so many things that can go wrong during the course of a career. One minute you can be playing in the first team and looking as though you have the world at your feet, and the next moment everything can change.

I experienced my first temporary halt to the good times at the beginning of April 1985 during a home game against Leicester which we won 3–1. I went up for a ball and landed awkwardly, but didn't really think I'd done anything worse than turn my ankle. I actually played on for a while but eventually had to come off, which is when I discovered that I'd broken my fibula. It was a real blow to me, because that was the first time I'd had a serious injury and the thought of not being able to play depressed me. The good thing was that the break happened towards the end of the season, so I only missed seven league games, but at the time it seemed like the worst thing in the world to me, and it meant that I saw a lot more of the physio's room than any foreign beach during that close season. Little did I know that it was the first of many tastes of the treatment table. I was to become all too familiar with it a few years later as a catalogue of niggling injuries began to blight my career. Still, my absence gave my mate George Lawrence a chance to have a decent run in the side. Although George had started with me at Southampton, he had been transferred to Oxford in 1982, but at the start of 1985 he returned to The Dell and was obviously keen to play first-team football and try to establish himself.

George wasn't the only arrival early that year, because Lawrie McMenemy also managed to bring in another player who was full of experience and skill – Jimmy Case from Brighton. Jimmy was 30 years old at the time and had won everything with Liverpool before heading south for Brighton. I'd watched him on TV playing for the Merseysiders and always thought he looked like a very effective midfielder. He could pass, tackle and shoot, and he had a great engine which allowed him to do an awful lot of work. But it wasn't until I played alongside him in the same team that I came to realise just how good he was. We seemed to hit it off instinctively on the pitch, and during the time we were both at the club we also hit it off away from the pitch. The two of us used to have some good nights out in Southampton, leaving Jenny and Jimmy's wife Lorna at home. We sometimes didn't manage to get back until the next morning. You can just imagine how that went down with the two girls, but it still didn't stop us doing it a few times. On the pitch Jimmy used to supply some great passes for me. What some people didn't know was that Jimmy had problems with his hearing, but the routine we got going meant that it wasn't necessary for us to shout to each other. I just used to widen my eyes when I wanted the ball played, and, believe it or not, Jimmy would literally wait until he saw the whites of my eyes before releasing it. His passes were usually inch-perfect and they certainly set up a few goals and scoring chances for me.

But, as I said, the big news at the club that year was Lawrie McMenemy's departure. He left a gaping hole. He'd been around for a long time and had been such a big part of Southampton that it was difficult to imagine the place without him. There were quite a few names touted as his replacement, and I think a lot of managers would have loved the job because the club had a reputation of being patient and supportive. The chairman and board weren't the sort of people to fire a manager if he didn't get instant success; they tended to back the man in charge and seemed to realise that you have to build teams. These days, of course, there seems to be a lot more pressure on the man in charge. Everyone wants their team to be winners, but the truth is that only a handful of sides win anything in a season.

That was the case then and it's still true now. But it often seems that managers are not given any time at all in the Premiership. I suppose the money involved in just staying in the Premier League puts much more pressure on a manager. Twenty years ago you wanted to win the league or a cup and get into Europe if you were a First Division team. Nobody wanted to get relegated, but if it happened it certainly wasn't the end of the world and there was a good chance that you would bounce back again, because a club usually kept its best players even if they went down. All that has changed now. Relegation from the Premier League can have a devastating effect on everyone connected with a club.

There didn't seem to be any obvious replacement for Lawrie already at the club. Coach Lew Chatterley was offered the job, but he decided to follow his boss to the north-east. In a move that surprised a lot of people, Chris Nicholl was given the chance to take over. I'd played with Chris when he was our regular centre-half, but he'd left a couple of years earlier to go to Grimsby as their player-assistant manager. It was obviously somewhere Southampton regarded as a good place to learn your trade in that respect, because Lawrie had been the Grimsby manager before taking over at The Dell. I liked Chris. He had a reputation in the media as being a bit dour, but I always found him to be good company, a guy with a great sense of humour. I had no problem being managed by someone I had played with and I knew he was a straight bloke who would treat his players in the right way.

Although we'd qualified for Europe by finishing fifth in the league, it was the year of the Heysel tragedy in Brussels at the European Cup final between Liverpool and Juventus, and as a result English clubs were banned from playing in European competition. It was obviously a blow to those teams that had qualified, particularly for a club like Southampton which always welcomed a bit of extra money alongside the glamour and excitement of playing in the UEFA Cup, but it was something we just had to accept and get on with. From a personal point of view I was just pleased to be over my injury by August and fit enough to be playing again. And I started that

1985/86 season in the first team with a new ambition: after playing well for England at youth and under-21 levels, I now wanted to try and force my way into the full squad. I was well aware that 1986 was a World Cup year and the best footballers from around the globe would be heading to Mexico come June. Of course I knew I was a bit down the pecking order because there were some good wingers around on the England scene, and with a player like John Barnes already well established in the team the most I could realistically hope for was to try and get myself into the squad. I was still only 21 and I realised I had my whole career in front of me, but it didn't stop me wanting to do as well as I could. In fact, to be honest, the England squad for the World Cup wasn't uppermost in my mind when the season started; as far as I was concerned, the main thing was to test the leg with some competitive football and show everybody that I was fully fit again.

There had been some great times both for the team and for me on a personal level over the last few years. I'd scored the goal of the season in March 1984 with an overhead kick during the 2–0 home win against Liverpool. I also scored our other goal in what was the first live televised match at The Dell. Things like that not only stick in your own memory but also in the minds of the public. I think the Southampton fans saw me as quite an exciting player, and I continued to get good publicity in the sports pages of the papers and on TV. But that 1985/86 season as a whole was a funny one for the club. After getting used to success in the league and being a top-six side, we began to struggle. We still had good players, but as a team we couldn't quite get it together any more. By the turn of the year we were scrabbling around trying to find some decent form, and we still hadn't won a game away from home. Thankfully, that didn't stop me from getting the chance to show what I could do with the full England squad.

As part of the build-up towards the World Cup finals, at the end of January England were due to play in an away friendly match with Egypt in Cairo. If I'm honest, I have to say that I probably wouldn't have got the call from manager Bobby Robson had it not been for the fact that there were some injuries, and some players, like John Barnes, Mark Chamberlain and Chris Waddle, had FA Cup commitments. It was a great opportunity for me and the perfect birthday present, because the match was due to be played just over a week after my 22nd birthday, but as much as I'd wanted it to happen I was still a bit surprised to be included. Once again it was a case of things happening early for me when it came to playing football. I'd made my league debut as a sixteen-year-old, I'd got into the Southampton first team on a regular basis when I was still a teenager, I'd represented England at various levels by the age of 21, and suddenly here I was with the chance to play a full international. Not for the first time in my career, it was like a dream come true.

When I actually joined up with the rest of the players at our hotel on the Sunday night before the midweek game, I have to admit I found the whole thing a bit frightening. I'd been away on international trips with the England under-21 side, but that was different because I was with players who were pretty much my own age and we were all trying to impress and show that we had a future at international level. But when you first walk into a room and see a bunch of established players who have been in the England team for years it can be a bit daunting, or at least it was for me. Luckily, I already knew Peter Shilton and Mark Wright from playing alongside them at Southampton, but seeing some of the others, like Ray Wilkins, Gary Lineker, Kenny Sansom and Peter Beardsley, was a bit overwhelming at first. Still, they made me feel at home straight away and I never once got the feeling that I was an outsider.

We flew to Cairo, and as well as training and preparing for the match we also did the tourist bit for the photographers, who wanted to get pictures of us in front of the pyramids for the papers back home. Needless to say, it was a great experience for me just to be involved. I'll never forget training with the squad for the first time because Bobby Robson unwittingly managed to have us all in fits of laughter. As I've mentioned, I think I owed my call-up in large part to the fact that some of the other wingers who were usually in the squad were injured or unavailable for the game. Two of them, John

Barnes and Mark Chamberlain, were black like me, and as Bobby took the session he was his usual vocal and enthusiastic self. The problem was that he kept calling me Barnesy or Mark. The other lads loved it, and despite all the giggling I still don't think Bobby realised what he'd done, although eventually he got to know who I was.

When I was told that I'd actually be playing, it was the icing on the cake. Getting the call was one of the best feelings I've ever had in football. The match itself wasn't particularly good, but it was memorable for me because I scored the third goal in our 4–0 win. Ray Wilkins played the ball out to Trevor Steven, and as the ball was crossed in I found myself on the edge of the Egyptian penalty box. I didn't really have any time to think about what I was going to do. Instinct took over, I flashed at it, hit the ball on the volley with the side of my foot, and it flew into the net. The scoreline was a bit flattering and we didn't get too much praise for the performance, but as far as I was concerned it was a great game and one I will never forget. The goal I scored wasn't the greatest I've ever put in the net, but once again the fact that it was for England on my debut means that I rank it up there with the best of them. I'd made the leap into the England team, and although I knew there were other, more established players to come back into the side I still thought I was in with a chance of making the squad for the World Cup.

How wrong I was. That game proved to be my one and only taste of football as a full England international. I never heard another word from Bobby Robson and I never made it into another England squad. I'm not saying that he was under any obligation to give me an explanation as to why I was never picked again, but I would have appreciated a bit of feedback on exactly why I was overlooked, even if it had come from the FA and not Bobby. It wasn't something that nagged away at me, but at the same time I'd be lying if I said I haven't thought about it during the years that have passed since that game in Cairo. Did he think I wasn't good enough? Did he not fancy me as a player? Or were there just too many options open to him? I just don't know. I was young enough at the time to think that I'd get another chance, even when the World Cup squad was announced and my name didn't feature. After all, when you're 22 years old there's no reason to think that your international career is over after one appearance and one goal, but that was how it turned out for me. A one-hit wonder. I'm sure I could have done well for my country if I'd been picked again at a later stage, but the chance never came. Perhaps I just suffered from the fact that in the 1980s and early 1990s there were a number of good English wingers around.

That season I also went close once again to realising one of my biggest ambitions when we reached the FA Cup semi-finals for the second time in three years. Two seasons earlier it had been against Everton; this time we took on their Merseyside rivals Liverpool. It was strange, because although our league form wasn't that good we fancied our chances in the cup, and I'd had the satisfaction of scoring the winning goal against my local club when I netted at The Den in a fifth-round replay to knock out Millwall. A lot started to be made of the fact that we might reach Wembley in what was the club's centenary year, but it just wasn't to be. We played Liverpool at White Hart Lane and had Mark Wright carried off before half-time with a broken fibula. It was a real blow for us; it also meant that the injury put poor Mark out of the World Cup. For the second time the match needed extra-time before the outcome was settled, with two Ian Rush goals. Once again we'd missed out. Once again I'd come within a whisker of playing in an FA Cup final. Given our depressing league form – we finished the season in fourteenth place with just 46 points – it was probably the first time I thought seriously about whether I would achieve anything big with Southampton.

I was still a young player, and I loved the club and its fans, but for the first time it struck me just how different the odds are of winning things if you are with one of the bigger clubs. Southampton had earned a reputation over the previous decade for being able to punch above their weight with successful campaigns in the league and FA Cup, but we were never going to be one of the big hitters when it came to winning trophies. Lawrie had worked a minor miracle to win the cup in 1976 with a 1–0 victory over Manchester United that put the club on the footballing map. He'd skilfully been able to blend teams together with a mixture of youth and experience, but the fact that he'd decided to leave Southampton was probably an indication that he felt we might have gone as far as we could.

As I said, when the 1986/87 season began I was still happy at the club. Early in 1986 I'd signed a new contract that ran for two and a half years to the summer of 1988, and my wages had improved again with a pay increase that gave me £400 per week, plus £100 for every first-team appearance. It was a lot of money, and I knew I was being well looked after financially by the club. But things were never quite the same after Lawrie went, which I suppose was only to be expected. On a personal level I got on well with Chris Nicholl, but whether that was true when it came to some of the other players I'm not sure. Early in 1987, for instance, Mark Dennis had a big bust-up with Chris and the episode ended with Mark having his contract terminated by the club. He moved on to Queens Park Rangers. It was clear that Chris wanted to change things, and he knew that the club once again had some good young players coming through the ranks. Two of them were my brothers Raymond and Rodney, another was a Geordie striker called Alan Shearer, and then there was a teenager from Guernsey who had ridiculous amounts of talent. His name was Matthew Le Tissier.

Ray and Rodney had moved in with Jenny and me after we'd bought our house in Midanbury. It seemed the logical thing to do, because at the time the two of them were apprentices in digs, just as I had been. This, of course, meant that Jen had four kids to look after. Thankfully, Jenny was brilliant about the whole thing. I'm not sure too many women would have been that happy about having their boyfriend's brothers move in, especially as she had a baby to look after as well. And in the autumn of 1986 the house became even more crowded when Jenny gave birth to a daughter we called Elisha. I was delighted to have another child, and this time I was at the birth at Guy's Hospital in London. She now had two children and three footballers to look after, including all the washing and feeding that went with it. It's fair to say that once again I probably didn't think too deeply about the consequences for Jenny, but she seemed to take the whole thing in her stride. She also had to put up with a bunch of my mates descending on us on a fairly regular basis whenever there were home games. I would take off with them after a match and Jenny would sometimes have some of her friends over and they would go out as well, leaving Rodney and Raymond as ready-made baby-sitters.

Matt Le Tissier was the first of this talented group of young kids to make a name for himself at The Dell: he came on as a substitute early in the 1986/87 season, played a few games at the end of the campaign, and immediately looked as though he belonged in the first team. In fact, it seemed as though he'd played there all his life. He was followed by Shearer, and during the 1987/88 season they were both joined by Rodney, who in his late teens showed he had the talent and ability to make it at the top. He finished the season with three full league games under his belt and a goal, as well as being named a dozen times as a substitute. It was great for Rod and another proud moment for our mum and dad, who now had two of their boys playing football in the First Division. It was a great achievement, and it wasn't too long before the Wallace brothers went one better, all three of us making history by appearing in the same Southampton first team together.

I'm glad that we got the chance to play together that day, for 1988/89 was my last full season at The Dell. Within a year of the Wallace brothers playing together for Southampton my long and happy association with the club would come to an end and I would be preparing to run out on to the field of play in the Theatre of Dreams.

CHAPTER SEVEN

MAKING THE RIGHT MOVE

It was either love, madness or a touch of both, but early in 1988 Jenny agreed to marry me. I can't claim I exactly swept her off her feet with the way I proposed; I remember only casually saying to her one day, 'I suppose we might as well get married.' The good thing for me was that she said yes, and we tied the knot at Southampton Register Office on 15 February. Time has proved that it was the right move for both of us. We were still only 24 at the time, but it seemed as though we'd known each other pretty much all our lives. We loved each other and we were best mates.

Jenny put up with an awful lot from me in those days and I've often wondered why she stuck it out and didn't just walk away. One of the reasons was that we had such a deep, strong bond. It sounds like a cliché, but in our case I honestly believe it's true: we're soul mates. We came from the same place, we experienced a lot of the same things, and for whatever reason there was a genuine attraction between us, even when we were just kids playing in the adventure park in South London. The fact that I was black and Jen was white never came into it. We just liked each other and had fun. When the time came for me to move down to Southampton it could have been the signal for us to pack in seeing each other, but that never happened. Sure we both saw other people during those early days, but had that not happened I doubt we would have stayed together. Although I played for a club that was nicknamed the Saints, I admit that I was anything but a saint in the way I treated Jenny so often in our relationship. Just to illustrate that point, I have to confess that on the night of our wedding I went out to a club with a few mates and left Jenny at home. It wasn't quite as bad as it sounds because she had some friends and family with her, but it certainly wasn't what you expect the groom to do on his first night as a married man. Luckily for me she put up with that little episode, along with all the others, and happily, despite all the problems we've had since, we're still together today. I genuinely feel blessed that Jen has been with me all this time. I don't think it's an exaggeration or being melodramatic to say that with all that has happened to me in more recent years, without her being there and caring for me I might easily have wound up dead.

Nobody can have any real idea of what is waiting for them down the line when they get married, and that was the same for us on that February day in 1988. What I did know was that we were a lot luckier and financially better off than many couples of our age who got married at that time. I was doing a job that I loved, and getting well paid for it. Most guys from my background would have given their right arm for the chance to do what I was doing, and although I was aware of that to some extent, it's also true to say that I probably took a lot of what was going on in my life for granted. Years later I had time and very good reason to reflect on the fact that I hadn't taken it all in and appreciated what I had then as much as I would have liked, but everyone knows that hindsight is a wonderful thing, and I was no different to a lot of people who just get on with their lives and forget just how good things are until the time comes when life is not so good any more.

Marrying Jenny was the right move for me on a personal level in 1988, and, with my current contract ending that summer, I also knew that I needed to start making the right move on a professional level as well. Ever since that semi-final defeat by Liverpool in 1986 I'd started to think about what life might be like at another club. It wasn't that I was unhappy at Southampton – in fact the opposite was true – but I did want to win trophies and further my career. I'm not saying things would have been different for me with regard to the World Cup in 1986 if I had been with a bigger club who were winning trophies, but I couldn't shake the nagging feeling that I needed to move on. Football at The Dell was still a lot of fun, though. I liked the players who were at the club, it was quite exciting to see the younger boys coming through just as I had only a few years earlier, and of course I had even more of an interest in what was happening because it involved members of my family.

Although Rodney was the striker and attracted more of the headlines, Raymond was also making steady progress and was turning into a solid prospect who could do a job in defence or in midfield. The great thing from their point of view was that they were at a club that was prepared to give its youngsters a chance. Lawrie had done that with me, and Chris Nicholl was no different in that respect. He moved into the manager's seat knowing exactly how the youth set-up was structured and also how successful it had been. He knew that he had to do the same sort of thing Lawrie had been so clever at, and mix experienced professionals with good young talent. He brought in the experienced defender Russell Osman from Leicester, and Neil Ruddock from Millwall, but Southampton simply didn't have the cash to compete in the transfer market with the big clubs and because of that they had to work a different route. It had borne fruit in the past, and after a year or two it was beginning to work for Chris, but there was no way I could afford to wait around for ever.

To many people, especially Southampton supporters, that is going to sound selfish, just another example of a footballer showing no loyalty. But you have to remember that even though I was only 24 I'd been with Southampton for a long time; it was almost nine years from the time I made my first-team debut to the day I played my last game in the team's colours. I don't think there is a single supporter who could look back on that period and point to a game where I didn't give everything. I admit it didn't always work out, and like any other player I had some poor games, but the one thing I could always guarantee fans was effort and commitment. My game was always based around attacking the opposition and taking players on, and I think supporters warm to a player like that. I certainly had a great time playing for the club, and to this day I have very fond memories of Southampton and its fans.

I think that by 1988 Chris and the club knew that I was thinking about what life would be like elsewhere, but at the same time they knew I genuinely loved Southampton. Being somewhere I felt comfortable and with people I liked meant an awful lot. I might not have caught Bobby Robson's eye again after that one international appearance against Egypt, but that didn't mean I wasn't still performing well at club level. There was quite a bit of talk about whether I would be on my way, with Arsenal mentioned as one of the teams who might be interested in signing me. I have to admit that I didn't do anything to stop the rumours, but I didn't start them either. I was in the prime of my career, and even though I was only 24 I had a lot of First Division experience behind me and had proved beyond doubt that I could perform at the top level. I was a winger, but I also scored goals. I had shown, too, that I could come inside and play as one of the main strikers if I was asked to. I'm not saying I was the greatest player in the world, but I do know that I was a good player, and a lot of teams in the First Division wouldn't have minded me being in their squad.

At the beginning of 1988, Southampton came up with a new deal. They had always treated me fairly, and for a club of their size they had managed to pay me well during the time I had been at The Dell. The last contract I had signed was for a basic wage of £400 a week with appearance money and bonuses on top; the new deal they offered was for two and a half years starting off at £500 a week and £150 for each first-team appearance, and the basic would then rise to £550 that summer and £600 a week a year later. There was also a lump-sum loyalty bonus of £20,000 due in the summer and two further bonuses of £10,000 each year for two years after that. In addition there would be quarterly wage bonuses of £1,300. It was a good deal, and a sign that they were serious about keeping me. In the absence of any concrete offer from another club, there seemed no reason for me not to agree to the contract. It wasn't as if I hated the place, and I decided that if I was going to move at some stage it would happen whether I'd signed a new contract or not. Until it did, I just wanted to keep on playing as well as I could for Southampton.

The 1987/88 season was another mediocre campaign for us, ending again in mid-table just as it had done in 1986/87, but we started 1988/89 brightly, and suddenly I wasn't the only Wallace on the team sheet every week. Rod had only started three league matches the previous season, but as I've already said, he was becoming part of the first-team set-up and was a substitute on quite a few occasions. Chris Nicholl had obviously liked what he saw because Rodney started the new season in the first team and remained there throughout. It was great having one of my kid brothers playing alongside me in the team, and he soon proved to be a hit with the fans, who took to him in the same way they had to me a few years earlier. And as I've already mentioned, it wasn't too long before the Southampton supporters were welcoming a third Wallace to the team. On 22 October Raymond lined up alongside Rodney and me for the home game with Sheffield Wednesday. We lost the match 2–1 but it was a brilliant day as far as the three of us were concerned, and the same applied to all our family and friends who were watching the game from the stands. It made a bit of history, because by fielding three brothers in the same team Southampton became the first league side to do so since the 1920s. Mum and Dad were understandably proud of the three of us. Dad actually got quoted in the *Echo*, the local Southampton paper. It was something I shall never forget, and I think it meant the world to the three of us. After the game we took our parents and other members of the family out for a meal in town to celebrate.

I still find it incredible that the three of us managed to make it through to that level of football with the same club, and it has to be said that Southampton's policy of playing youngsters if they thought they were good enough was a key factor. There were plenty of clubs the three of us could have gone to as kids, but I doubt whether any club but Southampton would have given us the chance to play First Division football together. That game helped Raymond to show what he could do, and he played a full part in the season, starting 25 league games – just two less than me. Rodney took the lion's share with 38 starts, and he scored a dozen goals as well, just to underline the fact that he had truly arrived in the First Division. His pace and eye for a goal shocked a few people in the division, but it didn't surprise me. I knew the kind of ability he had, and the same applied to Raymond.

Matt Le Tissier also blossomed that season, playing more than twenty games in the first team. It was a measure of his ability that he was often able to look as though he'd been a regular for years. If there is such a thing as a natural, then that description fitted Matt perfectly. He had the skill to turn a game, even at the age of twenty, and he could do outrageous things with the ball. He lacked pace, but his ability was enough to mark him out as someone very special. The thing I noticed most about him was how alive he became on the football field. Matt was an easy-going kid, not at all flash, perhaps the most unassuming player you could ever have come across. In the dressing room he'd be in the corner with his head down; he certainly wouldn't be the sort joining in all the banter and jokes. He was shy and wasn't the type to push himself forward, preferring instead to hang back and let the others do all the shouting and screaming. But once he was on the football field he was transformed. It wasn't that he became loud or boisterous, it was just that he looked totally in command of everything he did. He was self-assured, brave enough always to be looking for the ball no matter where on the pitch he was because he knew he had the ability to cope with situations other players wouldn't be able to deal with. I've seen him shoot from impossible angles and distances; I've seen him do things few other players would have attempted. But Matt believed in himself. He wasn't being flash, he was just being honest. In effect, it was like him saying, 'Look, if you give me the ball when I want it I'll create something for you.' Of course, it didn't come off for him all the time, but I suppose that's part of being a genius – the willingness to take the sort of risks others would never dare take, and not being afraid to fail. Certainly in the seasons that followed he probably did more than any other Southampton player to make sure they stayed up, often winning them games they had no right to win simply because he'd pulled something special out of the bag.

If Matt was a quiet and unassuming talent, the same certainly couldn't be said of the other youngster who was busy making a name for himself at the club. I don't think it would be wrong to describe Alan Shearer as flash – not in a nasty way, purely in a way that says, 'I know how good I am and I'm going to make it all the way to the top!' The club knew that they had a real goalscoring talent as soon as he joined. I remember watching him in youth games and being amazed at his power and strength. When he first played in the senior team he was only eighteen years old, and although he wasn't really that tall at five feet eleven inches, he seemed to win everything in the air. He loved scoring goals, and you could see a real belief in everything he did. Alan was the sort of forward who would frighten defenders because not only was he brave and willing to put himself where it hurts on a football pitch, he was also a lethal finisher with his head or his feet. Whoever was marking him knew they were in for a hard time because he was constantly on at them. He also had great control with the ball at his feet, and was very adept at shielding the ball from opponents and bringing others into play. When he didn't have the ball he'd snap at heels and tackle as if his life depended on it. It's something he's done throughout his career, and I think his willingness to work so hard throughout a game has been a big part of his success. He didn't actually go around saying he was going to play for England in those days, but it didn't surprise me when he made it because he was full of confidence. He was a strong personality. The fact that he was prepared to travel from one end of the country to the other and live in digs in Southampton shows just how much he wanted to succeed, and also gives an insight into the character of the man.

Alan, Matt, my brothers and a few other young players were the future for Southampton. As I watched them go from strength to strength I felt more than ever that it was the right time for me to move on. By the beginning of September 1989 I had put in no fewer than four transfer requests to the club. The club weren't very happy, and neither was Chris Nicholl. Not only did he want me to stay, he also didn't like the fact that my wish to leave had by now become very public. As well as Arsenal, there was talk of Chelsea, West Ham, Tottenham and Manchester United being interested. It was a situation that couldn't go on for ever.

With all the speculation flying around about a possible move I decided I needed the help of someone who knew the game and who I could trust to look after my interests in any deal. Bob Higgins had been a major influence on my career. He was the man I'd first met when Southampton signed me, and he'd been responsible for bringing a string of very good young players into the club, including my two brothers. As Southampton's development officer he was the person who first got to see any promising youngster, and he'd certainly done a great job for me. I'd always stayed in touch with him, and by this time he'd set up his own agency, the Bob Higgins Soccer Academy. I turned to Bob for advice and ended up signing a contract with him to act as my agent. It seemed the logical thing to do, and it took a lot of the pressure off me. If there were press enquiries to be answered I let Bob deal with them while I got on with the job of trying to play football.

I was told that Manchester United were showing more than just a passing interest in me and that they were willing to offer £750,000 as a transfer fee. It was a lot of money, but it was not enough as far as Southampton and Chris Nicholl were concerned, and they turned it down. It was a real blow to me at the time, because having a club like United come in for me was like a dream. As a player you often read transfer speculation about yourself, but until a bid is on the table or your club agrees to let you go it means very little. All the speculation until then had focused on me joining one of the big London clubs, and I suppose I'd thought that if I did move, it would be to the capital. Moving north and signing for Manchester United never really entered my head, but as soon as I heard about their offer I thought of very little else. I also believed that a move there would help my chances of getting back on to the England scene. It had been more than three years since I'd played against Egypt, and I thought that playing for a club like United would improve my chances of forcing my way back into the reckoning no end. What worried me was that I might have lost the chance because of Southampton's refusal to accept the offer, but happily for me, United were determined to buy me and they very quickly put in an increased bid of £1.2 million, which was an awful lot of money back then. It was enough to get Southampton to change their minds and accept the offer, leaving me free to negotiate personal terms with United.

The situation felt a little bit strange because I'd only ever been connected with one club during my entire professional footballing life, and Southampton wasn't just a club to me, it was like a family. But I'd made the decision that I wanted to leave that family and move away from the 'home' I'd known for so long, and it was up to me to deal with the emotions that went with that. What made the situation seem even stranger was the fact that it was United who were after me. They were the most glamorous club in Britain as far as I was concerned, and although at that time they weren't the force they have been in recent years, they were still massive. They also had Alex Ferguson as their manager, who had worked miracles with Aberdeen and broken the stranglehold Celtic and Rangers had on Scottish football by winning trophies including the European Cup Winners' Cup. He'd become one the hottest managers around, and big things were expected of him. His move to Old Trafford in 1986 to take over from Ron Atkinson hadn't been an instant success, and by the time he came in for me there were murmurings that Fergie was under a bit of pressure to deliver that season.

It was a reminder of the difference between somewhere like Southampton and a club like United. At the big clubs everyone expects and demands success; if they aren't competing for the title and winning trophies it is looked on as failure. If Southampton finished six or seventh in the league and had a decent run in one of the cups, most people would have said we'd had a good season. When we finished second and only missed out on the league by a few points in 1984 people in the football world couldn't really believe it. They couldn't quite understand how a club of our size and history could have done so well. As it happened, we had a good team with good players and a good manager in charge, so it wasn't such a surprise to us, but once again the reaction highlighted the fact that if you're a player and you want to win things on a regular basis, you have to be with a big club. The Premiership has changed football in this country, and people go on about how United, Arsenal and Chelsea have dominated things, but the truth is that has always been the case. The big clubs win the big prizes. Look at Liverpool in the seventies and eighties. Of course there are exceptions, usually in the cups – Southampton, Ipswich, West Ham and Wimbledon have all won the FA Cup as underdogs in the last 30 years – but in general the rule is that the big boys win the silverware.

By the time I got to talk to United I was 25 and had played nearly 300 games for Southampton. I was an experienced professional who had appeared at all levels of international football and I was the subject of a £1.2 million bid by one of the biggest clubs in the world. It should have helped my confidence as I travelled north, but although I was excited I was also nervous, just as I had been all those years ago when I first knew that Southampton were interested in signing me. However, having linked up with Bob Higgins, I was happy in the knowledge that he was going to be representing me in all the negotiations. Bob knew about football and he also knew me as a person. This wouldn't be just a case of an agent doing a deal and then walking away with his commission. I knew that Bob genuinely had my best interests at heart, and that when it came to the details of any contract he would make sure I wasn't sold short. This was a big move for me, and if I was going to do it and feel happy at my new club, Bob knew the sort of things that would be important to me.

These days having an agent is second nature to a player, but it wasn't quite the same back then. There were agents around, but not every player had one, as seems to be the case these days. If I was a young kid starting out with Southampton now, making my debut in the team as a sixteen-year-old, I'm sure everything would be very different. Theo Walcott broke my record for being the youngest ever player to appear in a Southampton first team when he played against Wolves in August 2005. He broke it by 171 days, and before the season was halfway through not only was there talk of a £10 million move, there were also reports of Theo and his 'advisers' sitting down with Saints officials to discuss his future. Just a matter of weeks later he was on his way to Arsenal in a deal that was worth around £12 million. It showed just how far the game has come in less than twenty years, and just what a different world it was for any young kid starting out in the game in the 1980s. I actually had the chance to meet Theo after he'd got into the Southampton team when the club asked me to do a video with him, because he'd just broken my youngest-debutant record. He seemed like a level-headed kid who was willing to listen and learn. If he stays like that I'm sure he's going to have a fantastic future in the game. But I had to smile when we met, because even then, after just a few games, there was talk of the big clubs being after him and it was clear he was very soon going to have to make a decision that I hadn't had to confront until nine years after I made my debut.

Bob and I travelled up to Manchester and went straight into a meeting with Alex Ferguson and the United chairman Martin Edwards. Bob went off with Edwards to talk over the contract details and I stayed with Alex as he outlined what he wanted from me and what his hopes and plans were for the club. I didn't really know too much about Fergie other than what I'd read in the newspapers or seen on TV, but from the moment I met him he seemed a pretty impressive figure. He was very self-assured, but at the same time warm towards me. Like Lawrie, he had a presence about him that let you know he was in charge, but he also came across as the sort of bloke you could communicate with. He was friendly, not at all aloof, and you could tell he had massive enthusiasm for the game and for United.

Just walking into Old Trafford was an experience in itself. Of course I'd been there over the years to play games for Southampton, and the ground had a special place in my memory as the venue of my surprise debut almost nine years earlier, but the thought of actually signing for them made this visit a bit special. I thought about all the great players they'd had at the club, and how I'd watched on TV as a kid and seen people like George Best skating across the Old Trafford pitch to score great goals. There was something about United and their red shirts that somehow seemed special and different to any other club. There was an aura surrounding them, and I think I picked up on that as soon as I went up there to talk about the move.

It was obvious to me that Alex was trying to build for the future, and he'd already brought several players to the club, including Paul Ince from West Ham who had only recently signed. There were, of course, already some good players there, and it was clear that Alex wanted to continue his activities in the transfer market. As I've said, there was pressure on him, but there was no sign of it as we chatted. Later, he gave me the grand tour of the ground. I'm sure he knew I was desperate to sign, but I left the ground that day without putting pen to paper, saying that I wanted to go back to Southampton and talk things over with Jenny. Alex and Martin Edwards were very relaxed about it. To be honest, pretty much everything had been agreed by the time we headed south again, though nothing had actually been signed.

If it was a big move for me, it was probably an even bigger move for Jen. Like me, she had never lived north of the Thames; now she faced the prospect of relocating to a part of the country she knew nothing about where her family and friends would be well over a hundred miles away. I remembered how Southampton had seemed so different for her when she first visited the place. I would be all right because most of my time would be spent playing football; Jenny was the one who would be left at home with two kids to look after in a strange environment. She was incredibly supportive when it came to me wanting to move away from Southampton. She realised why I had to get away and was prepared to go along with me, but I think at the back of both of our minds was the thought that it would be a London club and we could live in the capital, or at least close to it. Manchester had certainly never entered our thoughts when I started putting in transfer requests, probably because I believed they wouldn't be interested in me, but now the attractive offer on the table was from that neck of the woods. Although Southampton had pushed the boat out a bit with the last deal they had given me, they would certainly never have been able to compete with the sort of money United were offering. The contract was for four and a half years and the starting salary was £80,000 per year. Now I know some of United's current stars earn that in a week, but it was way more than I'd ever got in my life. There were also bonuses and a £150,000 signing-on fee, which was spread over four years. It was a different world in so many ways. I couldn't wait to join.

Thankfully, there weren't any long, agonising discussions with Jenny. She was just as keen as I was, and it was agreed that we would both travel up a couple of days later, on 16 September, to sign the contract and then watch United in their home game with Millwall. Jenny really liked Alex and felt happy about me joining the club. We were both aware of what a big move it was, but what also came across was that Fergie was keen on creating his own United family. Wives, girlfriends and kids were all part of the scene at the club on a match day, and I think we both immediately felt at home.

I was paraded on the pitch before the game as an announcement was made that I was the club's latest signing. Then I took my seat in the stands and looked on with the sense of anticipation a kid has on Christmas Eve. I'd just signed for Manchester United and I couldn't wait to start performing on one of the biggest stages in the game.

CHAPTER EIGHT

A CUP THAT CHEERS

One of the players in the United team against Millwall that mid-September afternoon was Paul Ince, and although I didn't realise it at the time, I was about to see a lot of Incy over the next few months. Like me, Paul was a London boy, and like me he had been a real favourite with the fans at the club he had come from. Of course that all changed once he joined United. We'd signed within a couple of days of each other, and because we'd only just moved to Manchester, the club put the two of us and our families into a hotel while we looked for houses. We were joined by another United new boy, big Gary Pallister, who had been bought from Middlesbrough.

It was a bit of a shock to the system for Jenny and me, but we soon settled into hotel life. The two of us plus the kids and our dog! It was certainly a different way of life for all of us, but it wasn't really fair on the dog, and we soon had to give him away to friends. Meanwhile, Incy, Pally and I began to get used to being part of Manchester United. We were all in the same boat really, because we'd come from smaller clubs where we had been very comfortable and had earned our reputations; now we all realised that we had to start again in many ways and prove we could do a job for United, and do it quickly. The fans were expecting big things from their new signings, and the club had spent a lot of money as Alex tried to put together a squad that could start to challenge for honours. I suppose there was pressure from the moment I signed for the club, but I never really felt it. I think that in terms of the media coverage we got, the focus was more on Fergie. We all knew he was in the spotlight; there seemed to be weekly talk about his job being on the line if United didn't deliver. To be fair to him you would never have guessed there was any pressure from the way he went about his job. He was always positive, always in control of things. He seemed like a man with a plan, and no matter what other people might have thought or said, he knew he was capable of producing a winning team.

For my part, I was desperate to show what I could do when I arrived. I wanted people to see that I could perform just as well, if not better, for United than I had done for Southampton. I got my first taste of life in a red shirt on 20 September 1989 in a Littlewoods Cup match at, of all places, Portsmouth. I was used to getting stick at Fratton Park whenever Southampton went there, and it was no different that night, but at least I had the satisfaction of scoring a goal. Incy got the other two as we ran out 3–2 winners. It was a good start for me, but it didn't take long for things to go pear-shaped. Three days after that win over Portsmouth we were thrashed 5–1 in a derby game against Manchester City. The knives were straight out for Fergie. Welcome to the big time. As if that wasn't bad enough, I very quickly picked up a hamstring injury, and instead of getting a decent run in the first team I found myself sitting on the sidelines. The hamstring was the first of quite a few I picked up during my time at Old Trafford. I'd also had them at Southampton, and I cursed my luck every time, but it was nothing compared to what was to come. I knew I was a good player, and Alex Ferguson must have thought the same otherwise he wouldn't have paid so much money for me, but at the same time I'm sure he must have wondered what he'd done because every time he saw me during those early few months I seemed to be having treatment. He was under pressure, the team weren't doing well on the pitch, and one of his new, expensive signings was sitting it out because he was struggling with his fitness. I'd had injuries at Southampton, but they'd been spread out during my time there. The trouble with my career at United was that from day one I seemed more often than not to be sidelined through no fault of my own. These minor but frequent injuries would blight my time at Old Trafford.

The fact that Jenny, me and the kids were in the Ramada hotel didn't help matters either. It's always nice to have your own place, but when you move from one end of the country to the other things like that take time. It wasn't horrible living in a hotel, and with Paul and Gary there for company it made things a lot more enjoyable. The three of us got on well, and Jenny got on with their girlfriends. It was nice for me to have a couple of team-mates on hand to chat with and pass the time. Incy, of course, was full of confidence from the very first day I met him, and he's never changed. He had the nickname 'The Guvnor' on the pitch, and it kind of summed up the way he played. He wasn't afraid to mix it with anyone, but at the same time he was some player as well. He had great ability, and as a midfielder he was always available and happy to get stuck in and win the ball. It was no surprise to see him go on and do so well, not only for United but also for clubs like Inter Milan, Liverpool and Middlesbrough – and, of course, for England. He's still doing a great job for Wolves. You won't get a more competitive player in the league because it's the only way he knows how to play. Pally was a much quieter character, but he too was to go on to become another really important figure at United. He was a big guy and great in the air, but he could play a bit as well and certainly wasn't the sort of central defender who just liked to whack the ball anywhere in the hope that it would find one of his players. He formed a great partnership with Steve Bruce, who was also a great player and a nice guy. The two of them were like a rock for United at the back, and I'm sure the fact that Fergie had probably the two best centre-backs in the country had a lot to do with the success the club enjoyed a few years down the line.

However, staying in a hotel wasn't the best thing that could have happened to me at that time. I was eating hotel food every day, and I suddenly began to put on a few extra pounds. We also used to have friends visiting most weekends, and I'm afraid the old hotel bar took a bit of a beating on occasion. The staff would fill it up and we would empty it. Both Jen and I liked a drink, and I'm sure that, coupled with all the food, contributed to the weight problems I began to have. It wasn't as if I put on a couple of stone or anything like it, but a few extra pounds made a difference to someone like me, especially as I wasn't training every week.

The fact that the move had happened relatively quickly meant that Jenny and I had hardly had time to think about some of the more basic things, like what we were going to do with our house back in Southampton. Buying and selling property is never easy, and with me busy at the club the burden of looking for a new house in the Manchester area fell to Jenny. My brothers, Raymond and Rodney, were still living with us in Southampton when we left, so they suggested renting our old house from us. They were both flying at Southampton while I was struggling with my fitness, and getting rave reviews for their performances. It was great to hear that they were doing so well, and I used to keep up with all the news and gossip by way of regular weekly phone calls to them, usually on a Friday so that I could wish them luck for the next day's game. The renting was a perfect arrangement because we knew the house was being looked after and the money helped to pay for the mortgage that we still had on the property. But Jen and I still needed to clear up some bits and pieces in Hampshire and decided to go back for a few days to sort things out.

I've already said that when I was at Southampton the fans were always really good to me. I think a few of them might have been a bit upset when I let it be known that I wanted to get away from the club, but the majority were sensible people who could see I had to do it for the sake of my career, and they appreciated what I'd done for the club. Nobody could have loved Southampton more than I did, and having come right through the ranks and stayed so long I think I proved my loyalty. But there comes a point in a footballer's life when he's with a club like the Saints when he has to ask himself if it's time to move on. To be honest, I was always surprised at Matt Le Tissier staying at The Dell when he could surely have moved to a bigger club. I know that at one point lots of people assumed he would go to Chelsea, but nothing happened. Matt decided that he was happy at Southampton, and there's certainly nothing wrong with that. It's just down to personal choice, and I think he's rightly earned a legendary place in the history of the club, not just because he resisted moving elsewhere, but because of the fact that he helped the club survive and stay in the Premiership on the back of some brilliant individual performances. In my case, I decided to take a different route, and even though things weren't working out immediately at United for me, there was no doubt in my mind that I would come good, and so would the team. Still, going back to Southampton to sort out personal bits and pieces felt a bit strange. Everything was familiar, but I wasn't as much part of the place as I had been when I was playing for the club only a short time earlier. And some locals, as I was about to find out, still felt bitter about my move to Old Trafford.

Jenny and I had always enjoyed going out in the area when we lived in Southampton, and one of our favourite haunts was the Indian Cottage restaurant. They did great food in there and they always made us very welcome, so one night during our visit we decided to go back there. Two of Jen's friends, Jo Mitchell and Kelly Saffery, came along as well. The three girls and I were shown to our table, and as soon as we went into the restaurant I could see that a couple of guys on another table had recognised me. It was no big deal as far as I was concerned; it had often happened in the past. People might say something and have a joke or ask for an autograph, but usually it was no more than that. There was a bit of banter as we ordered our food and I thought nothing more of it.

But then the mood started to change a bit. The two guys suddenly began to have a go about the money I was earning with United. It was clear they'd had a few drinks, and I could tell that things might start to turn nasty. Before long their comments were beginning to disrupt our meal, and a nasty atmosphere developed. All of a sudden, all hell broke loose. The two men began to go for us, with tables and food flying everywhere. It was like a scene from a Wild West movie. Luckily, I had my own gunslingers with me in the shape of Jen and her two mates, and none of them was afraid to get stuck in. I'd seen Jenny in action before, dishing out punishment in clubs to girls who she thought had gone a bit too far with me. She might have had the smile of an angel, but I knew from personal experience that it wasn't a good idea to cross her. She wasn't in the habit of taking nonsense from anyone. Quite literally, if push came to shove, she knew how to take care of herself. Sure enough, the girls swung into action quicker than I could say chicken vindaloo, and the two blokes didn't know what had hit them. In the end the four of us were swinging at the two of them as the rest of the customers looked on in total disbelief. We eventually got the better of them, and with the help of some of the waiters they were slung out of the restaurant. I think we somehow managed to finish our meal after all the commotion, and the restaurant staff were apologetic because they had seen what had gone on and knew that all we had done was defend ourselves. Mind you, I doubt they had ever seen three girls do what Jenny, Jo and Kelly did.

Things worked out all right for us that night and Jenny came out of it unscathed, but it brought to mind an incident years earlier when we had just started going out together. We'd been to the cinema and were walking home when we walked past a big guy who was walking the other way. Jen and I were only about fifteen at the time and suddenly the guy started shouting at us, racist stuff about me being black and her being white. Then I realised that he'd turned back and was coming after us. He went for me and swung a boot in my direction, but I managed to see it coming and ducked out of the way. Unfortunately, Jenny was standing directly behind me, and as I ducked she took the full force of the boot in her face. She ended up looking battered and bruised as the guy ran off, but typically she managed to joke about it, saying that next time she'd learn how to duck at the right time as well.

When I did get myself fit and back into the United side the pressure was really on. The team had underperformed, and as a result there was more speculation about Fergie's future. It's hard to imagine it now after all the success he's had at the club, but at the time there was a definite cloud hanging over the place, and Alex's ability as a manager was being questioned. He might have worked wonders with Aberdeen, but that counted for nothing when it came to United and their supporters. They wanted success, and at that stage in his Old Trafford career any sign of silverware seemed a long way off. To be honest, I think the pressure and expectation started to get to some of the players as well. Some of the performances bore all the familiar signs of a team playing without any real confidence. People weren't relaxed enough to try things during the course of a game; it was all about not making mistakes rather than trying to go at teams and open them up. As one of the new boys I was getting plenty of publicity, even when I was out of the side injured, but the truth was that my dream move was turning into a bit of a nightmare.

One of the great things about the English season, however, is that even if a team is having a bad time in the league, the FA Cup can often offer you a hand and turn your fortunes around. A win in the cup can suddenly give a losing side some belief in themselves, and they begin to pick up a bit of form. It doesn't matter that for most of the first half of the season they may have been under the cosh, a win in the third round can give a side new focus. By the time January 1990 came around, the FA Cup offered all of us the chance to put a new complexion on a season which had been such a disappointment. The away draw at Nottingham Forest not only gave us a break from the league, it was also a chance to do something positive with our season. Once again there was talk of Fergie losing his job if we didn't win at the City Ground. Despite the gossip, I don't think the players felt they were under any greater pressure. We'd had criticism right through the season for our performances, and we knew we just had to get on with things and hope that we came through the tie.

It's strange to think now of just how significant that game was, not just to the manager but also to the club. When the final whistle blew that day a Mark Robins goal for us was enough to separate the two sides and put us in the hat for the next round. The win that day changed an awful lot of things. Whether or not Fergie breathed a sigh of relief I don't know, but I do know that it gave everyone at the club a lift. It wasn't an end to the doom and gloom merchants, but it gave us something to aim for. The FA Cup was one of the three big domestic trophies, and because of its history there was always something special about playing in it. One of the reasons I'd wanted to move was to play in an FA Cup final. I'd gone close on two occasions with Southampton, but I felt that joining a club like Manchester United would give me a better chance of walking out on to the Wembley turf. Beating Forest was only one step, but it was a step in the right direction.

We went to Hereford in the next round and recorded another 1–0 win thanks to a Clayton Blackmore goal, and then, on 18 February, had a really tricky draw away to Newcastle in the fifth round. On the morning of the game I woke up to find a story in the paper claiming that I could be on my way out of Old Trafford if we lost the match against Newcastle. The article said that my move hadn't worked out and that Fergie was ready to use me as part of a package to tempt striker Tony Cascarino from Millwall. I'd only been a United player for five months, Jen and I had only just moved into a brand-new house we'd bought in Worsley, and they were already saying that I might have to pack my bags! I knew I hadn't exactly set the place on fire, but that was due mainly to the fact that I'd had injuries. I needed a steady run of games under my belt if I was going to show everyone at United exactly what I could do. It's not the sort of thing you want to read on the day of a match, particularly an important cup game, but I just had to put it out of my mind. Happily, it didn't affect my game and I managed to score one of our goals in a 3–2 win, Mark Robins and Brian McClair getting the others for us. Suddenly we really were in with a chance because it was now down to the last eight, but the pressure was still on us as we prepared for the sixth round. So far all of our games had been away from Old Trafford, and the trend continued when we were drawn to go to Bramall Lane and face Sheffield United.

In these early months of 1990 we still weren't exactly covering ourselves in glory when it came to the league. In fact, we were hovering around the wrong end of the table. It seemed as though every time United were mentioned in the press, the statistic that the team had been assembled for £13 million was also in there somewhere. We were the expensive side that had failed to deliver, and it was looking more and more likely that if we were going to justify that spending it would be in the FA Cup, particularly after a Brian McClair goal in the 29th minute of the game in Sheffield meant that we found ourselves just one match away from the final.

Quite often when people look at a team's run in a competition they will utter the old football cliché and say, 'Their name must be on the cup.' I think a few started to say exactly that after the draw for the semi-finals was made and we were paired with Oldham, the only team left in the competition from outside the top division. Liverpool were due to play newly promoted Palace in the other semi-final and were expected to beat them, leaving the way clear for a titanic clash with us at Wembley. But football is never as easy or as predictable as people think, and cup football has always had a history of upsets, which is what makes it so interesting and exciting for the fans. Palace came out on top in a seven-goal thriller at Villa Park, and our tie turned into a six-goal thriller.

Oldham had already surprised a lot of people that season by getting to the Littlewoods Cup final and losing by the only goal of the game to Forest, so we knew that they certainly weren't going to be pushovers. The match also had the added spice of being a bit of a local derby, so it was decided that the best venue for our semi-final would be Manchester City's Maine Road. The game was probably everything the neutral would have wanted from an FA Cup semi-final, but for both sets of supporters I'm sure it was torture. It ended 3–3. I came off the bench to get our third in extra-time and put us ahead, only for Roger Palmer to equalise for Oldham and force the game into a replay. We met again three days later, and once again it was a nail-biter. I crossed the ball for Brian McClair to open the scoring for us, but Andy Ritchie got Oldham back on level terms and it needed an extra-time goal from Mark Robins to book a place against Palace at Wembley on 12 May. I found out later that it would be United's sixth cup final appearance in fourteen years, and despite the struggles of the season we were immediately installed as favourites to win. I was about to get the chance of realising one of my childhood ambitions by playing at Wembley, and for the first time since arriving at the club I began to relax and look forward to the big day.

The build-up to the final was everything I expected it to be. An awful lot of attention seemed to be focused on the match. Once again there was pressure on us because we were the favourites, and that meant there was pressure on Fergie as well. This was his chance to claim his first trophy as United manager, and considering all the talk there had been during the course of the season about him and the possibility of losing his job, I'm sure he was aware of just how much it meant. But once again you'd have been hard pressed to recognise that fact the way he carried on. It's probably something that all the best managers have: they are able to operate and concentrate even when things are pretty intense. I think Alex genuinely looked forward to that final, just like the rest of us; we all knew it was a chance to stamp our mark on things and prove that we weren't expensive flops.

There was all the usual pre-final stuff in the week leading up to the match, including being measured up for the cup final suits all sides seem to have. The wives and girlfriends got in on the act as well: they went out in Manchester to choose outfits to wear for the final itself and the reception afterwards. Jenny chose an elegant dress for the evening, but couldn't be bothered to get too dressed up for the match. She wore a denim jacket at Wembley – smart but practical, and typical of her. She wasn't really into flashy clothes or designer gear. She liked good-quality stuff but wasn't the kind of girl you could describe as ever getting caught up in the Footballers' Wives bit.

Any cup final is a big occasion for the teams involved, but considering the size of the club and its history there was no doubt United were more used to the big occasion than our opponents. Palace had done brilliantly to reach Wembley after just one season in the top flight, and they had a team who really worked hard for each other. Their manager, Steve Coppell, had been a great player with Manchester United and he'd done a good job since taking over at Selhurst Park six years earlier. They had some decent players in their side too, and none of them posed more of a threat than Ian Wright. It was strange to think back to the days when we'd played together in the same Sunday team, but it was no surprise to me to see him doing so well in the professional game, and at that time he was really beginning to earn a reputation for himself after proving he could score goals at the very top, just as he had done at any level he'd played in as a footballer. Wrighty had formed a lethal partnership with Mark Bright, and the two of them were a real handful for any team. But poor Ian had broken a leg a couple of months earlier and was injured during the run-up to the final, which meant that as we lined up for the kick-off on the big day he could only manage a place on the bench. I felt sorry for him, because I knew just how much it would have meant to him to start an FA Cup final; but I have to admit that as a team we were relieved that he wasn't lining up alongside Brighty.

It's quite often the case that after all the publicity and all the hype, finals turn out to be quite dull affairs leaving everyone wondering what the fuss was about in the first place, but that certainly couldn't have been said about our game with Palace. On paper we had the better, more experienced side, with the likes of Steve Bruce, Gary Pallister, Neil Webb, Mark Hughes, Paul Ince and, of course, the skipper, Bryan Robson, who had done a brilliant job since signing for the club in 1981. He'd also already lifted the FA Cup on two previous occasions with United and was desperate to make it a hat-trick. But pretty much from the first whistle both sides were committed, and there was a tremendous pace to the game. I think everyone watching the match got value for money.

We got off to a bad start, and I'm afraid I had a hand, or rather a foot, in it. I've never been the greatest defender or tackler in the game, and it was my mistimed challenge on Andy Gray that gave Palace a free-kick on the right. When the ball was played in, Garry O'Reilly got his head to it and put them in front. The good thing was that we got back into the game in the first half, and happily for me I managed to win the ball back and help set up the move that saw Bryan Robson score the equaliser. Mark Hughes put us in front after the break, and with about twenty minutes of the match remaining it looked as though we would hold on for the win, because Palace weren't really causing us any great problems during that period. But then a certain Ian Wright got the chance he had been waiting for.

Steve Coppell decided to bring Wrighty on as a last throw of the dice, and it soon became apparent that it was a gamble worth taking.

He had only been on the pitch for about three minutes when he showed just what a lethal finisher he was by cutting inside Gary Pallister in the penalty box and guiding a shot over the line to level the scores and set up a period of extra-time. And just to prove the first goal was no fluke, Ian got a second only a few minutes into the first period to put Palace in front again and turn the game upside down. It was a real shock to the system and a test for us as a team. We finished the first period with them still leading the game, but then proved that we had spirit and determination, whose presence some people doubted, by coming back with a third goal of our own. It was particularly satisfying for me because I provided the pass for Mark Hughes to go on and score.

The drawn game left everyone with a bit of a feeling of anti-climax. As a team we were pleased to have forced a replay, but at the same time part of me couldn't help feeling upset at the fact that we'd let them back into the match when it looked as though we had the game won. Overall, however, I was just pleased to have played in the final. It was a fantastic experience and it lived up to everything I'd hoped for, but it was a strange feeling to come off the pitch and still not have a result. It meant that the two teams had to meet again five days later, and having gone so close to lifting the cup I think we were all determined not to make any mistakes the second time around.

We were still favourites for the replay, but we certainly weren't arrogant or complacent. We knew that Palace had the ability to score, and that they would never say die. Fergie also showed how ruthless he could be when it came to team selection and dropped goalkeeper Jim Leighton, who had played for him at Aberdeen as well, in favour of Les Sealey. Jim hadn't had the best of games in the first match and it was clear Alex wasn't prepared to take the risk of hoping he would be better in the replay.

The first game had been quite an open affair with both sides doing a lot of attacking and producing plenty of goalmouth action, but the replay could not have been more different. I think Palace had clearly decided to make sure they tightened things up more, and it was certainly a more physical game that wasn't as exciting for the fans. I remember getting clattered a couple of times early on by the Palace defender Richard Shaw, and I knew I was in for a tough night. It was goalless at the break and seemed to be the sort of game that might be settled by the team that scored first. I think there was a lot more tension around than there had been in the first match, but there was no doubt that we had the edge, and in the second half we got the vital breakthrough when Lee Martin crashed in a shot from about sixteen yards out. This time there was no comeback from Palace, and when the final whistle blew it was one of the most magical moments of my life. Suddenly I remembered all those years I'd spent watching other players react to winning a cup final at Wembley. It was almost unreal for a second or two because now that I was in their position I wasn't quite sure what to do! That feeling soon went, though, and the sheer happiness and emotion of it all took over. There seemed to be players hugging each other all over the pitch, and all I could hear were our fans cheering and singing. I was a winner, and no matter what else happened to me in my career nobody would ever be able to take that away from me.

CHAPTER NINE

FERGIE'S FAMILY

I didn't know it at the time, but that Wembley final win proved to be the highlight of my Manchester United career. When I look back on my time at Old Trafford I have to say that my first season was probably my best. At least I played a number of games and was always in and around the first team, despite the little injuries I picked up. I also managed to show the United fans a glimpse of the Danny Wallace Saints supporters had come to know. I had some good games, particularly in the cup run, like the game at Newcastle where I not only played well but scored a good goal too. But I would be the first to admit that the move had not gone entirely as I had hoped. I had never really got going, and it seemed as though if I took a step forward, I would immediately take two steps back. It became a familiar theme of my time at United, and a big regret.

Of course, now I can look back with hindsight and start to understand and piece together what was going on. I honestly believe that during that 1989/90 season with United, I not only experienced my first taste of glory by winning the FA Cup, I also experienced my first taste of multiple sclerosis. Like any other player I had my ups and downs with form, but the fact was that during my time at Southampton one of my main assets as a player was my ability to turn in consistent displays for the club. I might have had a few stinkers on the pitch, but most people who saw me play will tell you that I could always be relied on, and that I always did my bit for the cause. At United, that changed. I think it was partly down to me feeling a bit more pressure than I had been used to, but the injuries and problems with fitness didn't help.

119

Southampton was the small club trying to live with the big boys, and consistently overachieving when you look at the size and set-up of the place. For quite a few years I had been one of the big fish in this lake, then suddenly, after joining United, it felt as though I'd swapped the lake for the ocean. I'd prepared myself for joining one of the biggest clubs in the world, but no matter how many times you go over things in your mind and think about the changes that are going to happen in your life after a big move, you can never fully understand what it's like until you start playing. I still think things wouldn't have been as bad if I had been able to get a good run of games under my belt from the very first day I signed, but it didn't happen like that. Instead, I got injured and it was stop-start all the way after that. At the time I just felt frustrated and put it down to a run of bad luck. It's something that can happen to a player. Having got away pretty much injury-free for a large part of my career I just had to accept that I had hit a bad patch; all I could do was make sure I worked my way through it.

The injuries mainly fell into three categories: they affected my back, groin or hamstring, and most of them seemed to occur down the right side of my body. It wasn't as if they all came at once, but it seemed as though I would pick up a niggle during a game or in training and be out of the reckoning for a week or two, come back and get fit, play a few games, then just when I thought I was getting my form and fitness again another injury would crop up and I'd be back on the treatment table.

If it was frustrating for me, then I'm sure it was just as bad for Alex Ferguson. Remember, he'd paid £1.2 million for me at a time when he was under pressure to produce a winning side and there were questions being asked about whether he should continue as United manager. It couldn't have been too heartening for him to turn up for training every morning and see one of his expensive signings missing again through injury. I wanted Fergie to see me flying on the training field and showing the sort of form I'd had at Southampton. Instead, the only reports of what I was doing came from our physio, Jimmy McGregor. I'd been bought to provide the sort of service players like Brian McClair and Mark Hughes would thrive on, but for a lot of the time the team had to make do without me. Managers live and die by results, and Fergie was no different. I wanted to be part of things and play regular first-team football, but it never quite happened.

The good thing was that at least the season ended on a high both for United and for me. The Wembley win was just about the best thing that had happened to me in football, and once we had won the cup and I'd been presented with my medal all the frustration that had been a big part of the season for me seemed to disappear. I'd ended it as a winner and achieved what I'd hoped for when I joined United. As we all celebrated that night I couldn't help feeling that the cup was going to be the first of many such occasions for me. I felt that once we'd cracked it by winning something we had the players and resources to build on the achievement. Time has proved that I was right in thinking that, but the bit I got wrong was that I thought I'd be playing a full part in it all.

The celebrations were tremendous after winning that night. We travelled back and had a full civic reception the next day, and suddenly everything seemed different. From being the heavily criticised team under the microscope we were now FA Cup winners with a place in Europe to look forward to in 1990/91, and people were talking about us in a completely different way. It was only one game, but it had far-reaching consequences for the club. It's strange to think of the way things might have gone for United in the 1990s had Palace managed to hang on at 3–2 in that first match. Fergie may well have been sacked, and where would United have gone from there? They say that one game can turn a season; well, perhaps it's true to say that in United's case one game turned the fortunes of the club for years to come.

I think Jenny was as thrilled as I was with the win. She never was and never will be a football fan, of course. She's never been the least bit interested in the game, though she used to go to matches and watch me, often having to bite her lip on occasion when fans were giving me stick from the stands. Mind you, I think she let a few of them know exactly how she felt a couple of times during my career as well. Jenny's not the sort to hold back, and although she realised that not every fan was going to like me, and having paid their money they had a right to voice their opinions, I think the time when someone called for Fergie to 'Get the little black bastard off' was a bit too much for her to take. 'That's my little black bastard you're talking about,' she shouted at him, 'so why don't you shut up?' I think it had the desired effect. As I said, she was really proud of me after that Wembley win because she knew just how much it meant to me. For a time she actually wore the medal around her neck on a chain. I loved seeing her wearing it. Jen and I went back a long way, and as kids I know I must have bored her with stories of how one day I'd be one of those players in a team that won the FA Cup. I knew that Ian Wright had had the same sort of dreams and I realised just how upset and depressed he would have been at losing out, especially as he had only been able to be part of it all as one of the substitutes. But you didn't have to be a football expert to know that his time would come again. Everyone knew Ian was destined for bigger things, and nobody could have been more pleased than I was to see him go on and become one of the best strikers the modern game has known.

Jenny and I used the summer break to settle properly into our new house. The months of living in a hotel had been fine, but when we actually moved into our own home I think it kind of marked a new chapter in our relationship. For the first time both of us felt like we were a proper family – Jenny, Remi, Elisha and me. Until then it had all been a bit different. In Southampton we had Rodney and Raymond staying with us and a constant stream of friends coming down to visit. Once we moved into the new house we felt as though we were on our own more and we began to carve out a new life in a new environment. We soon found new schools for the kids and it was nice for them to come home to a house instead of a hotel room. We also began to make new friends in the area. There weren't really any of the United boys who lived near us, because they tended to live on the other side of Manchester, but that didn't bother us. We would occasionally see them if someone was having a dinner or party at their house, but other than that we were satisfied with our new friends in the area and the occasional visit from our old friends from London and Southampton.

I've already mentioned that one of the consequences of living in the hotel for so long was that I put on a few extra pounds which I found hard to shift during the course of the season. After the cup win, and with all the problems I'd had with injuries and form, I decided that I would really work at getting myself in shape for the start of the new season. I wanted to hit the ground running and make sure that I didn't let myself down. I'd had enough of being out of the side; in 1990/91 I wanted to play a full part in things, domestically and on the continent, and let Fergie know that his money had been well spent.

The longer I spent at United, the more I got the feeling that Alex Ferguson was a similar character in many ways to Lawrie McMenemy. When I'd signed for United Alex had outlined his plans and it was clear he was in it for the long term. He wanted to build from the grassroots up, and make sure United was equipped to become English football's top club. United might have been massive, but one of the things that struck me from the very first time I spoke to him was the way he seemed to want to create a family within that club. He wasn't just interested in the big picture; the little things concerned him as well. Of course his number one priority was to win matches, but he paid a lot of attention to detail and also to what was going on at the club. He was well aware, for instance, that United had a great future in the offing with some of the kids who were coming through the ranks. As far as he was concerned, it wasn't just about the first team and nothing else. He made it his business to know what was happening at the club, and would watch reserve and youth games. The players had a lot of respect for him, and there was never any question that he was in charge or that things should be done differently, even when people on the outside were questioning his management. When I was struggling in those first few months he tried to ease my worries by sitting me down for a chat and telling me to relax a little and not worry about the fact that I was now playing for a big club like United. 'I bought you because of the way you played for Southampton, Danny, and all I want is for you to do the same here,' he told me.

I knew that what he was saying was true, but at the same time I realised that I only had a relatively short period of time to prove myself to him. A manager can't wait around too long for one of his players to hit form. He has to pick the best eleven he has for a game, and if that means you miss out because of your form or injuries then it's tough luck. I understood that, and that's why I was determined to try to give myself a bit of an edge when the players returned in early July for pre-season training. I did a lot of running and felt really fit by the time we all reported back to The Cliff, United's training ground. In fact, I'd lost about ten pounds in weight and felt a lot better for it. A big part of my game was based on pace and speed. Although I hadn't exactly felt heavy towards the end of 1989/90, I knew that I wanted to come back lighter, and I think Alex and his assistant, Archie Knox, were pleased with the effort I'd put in when the time came for the players to jump on the scales.

There was a good spirit during pre-season training, for two reasons. I'd played in Europe with Southampton and always enjoyed the trips we had during the time we were finishing high enough in the league to qualify. Being involved in an international club competition always adds something to a season, gives it an extra bit of spice, and the excited anticipation could be felt that summer at The Cliff. Secondly, all the players were aware that we'd removed the burden of not winning a trophy, though at the same time we'd raised expectations as well. It was up to us to get some more silverware soon, and the perfect place to start for us was the Charity Shield game against Liverpool a week before the new season. Once again it was an opportunity for me to play at Wembley, which made it my third appearance there since joining United. But unlike the FA Cup final replay this game didn't have a happy ending for me.

First of all we drew the match 1–1, which meant both teams got to keep the Shield for six months of the year, but on a personal note the game was a nightmare for me. After all the time, effort and hard work

I'd put in during the summer to make sure I came back fighting fit and ready to play in the first team, I managed to strain my groin during the game and had to come off. It wasn't the happiest way to leave the Wembley pitch, and more importantly it meant that I missed the start of the new season. To use a favourite footballing phrase, I felt absolutely gutted. I began to think my United career was jinxed. I'd had a bucketful of silly little injuries during the previous season and just wanted to make a fresh start. Missing the big kick-off was so disappointing after all the work I'd done. I knew I was really fit and strong. But instead of big crowds and nice green pitches, all I had to look forward to was the all too familiar surroundings of the treatment room.

Being injured and having to get yourself back to full fitness away from the rest of the team is a miserable experience, but there's very little you can do about it except get on with what the medical staff tell you to do and not complain. The worst part is that you find yourself on the outside looking in as far as the first team is concerned, and it's not a pleasant experience. I could feel myself slipping down the pecking order day by day, and there was very little I could do about it. It felt as though my career was passing me by. By the beginning of November I had started just one first-team game, and that was a European Cup Winners' Cup tie against Wrexham. It was hardly the sort of start to the season I'd hoped for.

I went to see Alex Ferguson about the situation and again he told me not to be so anxious and to try to relax a little more. He said that if I kept myself fit and involved my chance would come, and then it was up to me to grab it and make the most of the opportunity. I told him how frustrating it had been for me and that the little injury problems hadn't helped, which of course he knew already, but I needed to get the whole thing off my chest and make sure that he understood I was desperate to produce the sort of form that had made him buy me in the first place.

Happily, soon after talking to him I got the chance I'd been waiting for. Ironically, it was against Palace, though this time in the league. Although they'd flirted with relegation the previous season and been beaten by us at Wembley, they had started 1990/91 in great form, and when they turned up at Old Trafford they were protecting an unbeaten start. It turned out to be one of those games where pretty much everything I did went right, and it gave me a much-needed boost. We won the match 2–0, and I made one goal and scored the other. It couldn't have been much better, and after the match I got some great publicity along the lines of this being the match where Danny Wallace put his nightmare year behind him. I allowed myself to think that the Palace game was the opportunity I'd been waiting for for a fresh start, but perhaps I should have known better. I played in a few games after that, but the niggles resurfaced in December and I finished the year worrying about whether or not my knee would need an operation.

United were going well in the Rumbelows (League) Cup at the time – we'd already knocked Liverpool and Arsenal out of the competition, scoring nine goals in the process – and I was desperately hoping to make it back for the mid-January tie at The Dell with Southampton, but I had to pull out of it. The club sent me to a specialist to have the knee looked at. I feared the worse and thought I was going to have to have a cartilage operation. Luckily it was diagnosed as only being bruised, but the good news was short-lived. I might have avoided having an operation, but I went on to re-play the previous season, unable to really stake a claim to a first-team place. United went on to reach the Rumbelows Cup final, but this time, instead of being part of the team that walked out on to the famous Wembley turf that April, I watched the game from the stands. Sheffield Wednesday ran out 1–0 winners. It was a strange experience being back there just eleven months after the place had provided one of the happiest moments in my life. What a difference less than a year makes.

It was a miserable time for me. All the great hopes I'd harboured at the start of the season had been blown out of the water yet again. The really frustrating thing was that when I did get myself fit and back into action, I just wasn't performing at the level I wanted. I spent more time in the reserves than in the first team, and by the time the season drew to a close I'd played in just thirteen league matches.

Still, I was pleased for the team, who managed a second final that year, this time disputing the Cup Winners' Cup with Barcelona at the Feyenoord stadium in Rotterdam. My involvement in United's European campaign to this point had been confined to the substitutes' bench and a couple of brief appearances, so I didn't really expect to be part of things for the final. In addition, the match was due to take place on a Wednesday evening in mid-May and by this time the team pretty much picked itself; it was only a matter of who would fill the places on the bench. Fergie decided that I should be one of the substitutes. He could have picked his son Darren, who had made his United debut a few months earlier and was a solid midfielder who could operate on the right, but Alex must have thought I would be the better option in the circumstances.

So, on the Monday before the game I reported to Old Trafford for the coach trip to Manchester airport and the short flight over to Holland. We were all confident of winning the cup even though it meant beating the mighty Barcelona. The team had played well in Europe and the Cup Winners' Cup was our last chance to end the season with a trophy. Wednesday, of course, had won the League Cup, and Arsenal and Tottenham had already secured the league championship and the FA Cup respectively.

The atmosphere at the game was brilliant. Even as one of the substitutes I couldn't help being caught up in it. I would have loved to start the game, but I knew that was unrealistic and that once again I had to concentrate all my energies on the next season. We won the match 2–1, but had to hang on for the last ten minutes of the game. Both of our goals came from Mark Hughes, who scored after 68 and 74 minutes against one of his old clubs. But then, six minutes after Mark's second, Ronald Koeman got one back for the Spanish side, and it was nail-biting stuff until we heard the final whistle. There were the usual celebrations, naturally. Neil Webb was part of the squad that travelled to Holland for the game and he happened to be friends with the singer Mick Hucknall from Simply Red, who was a big United fan and was there at the post-match party. I recognised him, and Webby called me over to say hello. The celebrations were in full swing when suddenly a joint was produced and lit up. So there I was with Neil and Mick having a few puffs to help celebrate United's Cup Winners' Cup win over Barcelona. It was the first time I'd ever tried the stuff and I never thought I would ever do it again, but as things turned out I would use it again, though only for medicinal purposes.

Although as a member of the cup-winning squad I was present at the celebrations, unlike a year earlier when I had felt a real part of everything, this time it was different. I'd only played a bit part, and although I picked up a winner's medal I could hardly call myself a regular fixture of the winning team. I tried to join in as best I could, but it felt a bit weird. I was there on the pitch when all the pictures were being taken, but in many ways my mind was somewhere else. In the space of two years I'd gone from being one of the best young players in the country to someone who hardly got a game any more. For virtually my entire career at Southampton I was an automatic choice. I realised when I joined United that things wouldn't be the same and it wasn't going to be as easy for me, but at the same time I had a lot of confidence in my own ability and I knew that Alex Ferguson thought I could do a job for him. But after two full seasons the only direction I had gone in was backwards.

Just to add to my problems, United now had other options in my position. They already had Lee Sharpe and had brought in Andrei Kanchelskis, but there was also a gifted seventeen-year-old young-ster called Ryan Giggs who was making a name for himself. It was evident to anyone who saw him play that he was going to be a big star, and it was going to be a case of sooner rather than later. Ryan had it all. He was another one of those kids who immediately com-manded respect from the older players because they could see how much natural ability he had. So as I prepared for the new season in the summer of 1991 I knew I not only had to stay fit, I also had to try and regain top spot in the pecking order. With Lee, Andrei and Ryan around, that wasn't going to be easy. And Giggs, of course, was only

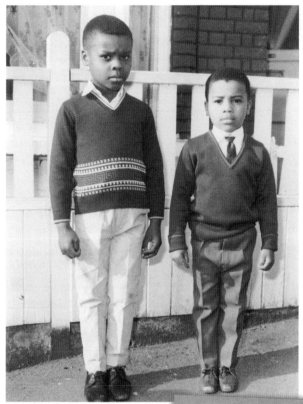

Clive (left) and me looking the picture of innocence. I was five years old.

The Schoolboy Penalty Competition

Today we continue at half time the extremely popular schoolboy penalty competition, sponsored by the South London & Kentish Mercury, and organised by the Millwall Football Club. The match today sees the quarter-finals of the under sixteen section. We would ask you to give the lads your support and encouragement, and to refrain from endeavouring to put a particular boy off, if his face is not to your liking.

RULES: Each boy will take three penalties, the one scoring the highest number will be adjudged the winner. In the event of a draw, each boy will take penalties alternately until a winner is forthcoming. In the event of time running out the competition will be continued at a date and venue agreed by the organisers.
In all cases the decision of the organisers is final.

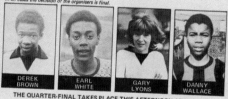

DEREK BROWN   EARL WHITE   GARY LYONS   DANNY WALLACE

THE QUARTER-FINAL TAKES PLACE THIS AFTERNOON AT HALF TIME AND THE LINE UP FOR THE KICKS WILL BE AS FOLLOWS:

UNDER 16 AGE GROUP

NAME	SCHOOL	COLOURS	1	2	3	TOTAL
GARY LYONS	CROWN WOOD	All White				
DANNY WALLACE	WEST GREENWICH	Black and Red Shirt Black Shorts				

UNDER 16 AGE GROUP

NAME	SCHOOL	COLOURS	1	2	3	TOTAL
DEREK BROWN	SAMUEL PEPYS	Yellow Shirt Black Shorts				
EARL WHITE	PECKHAM MANOR	Amber & Black Stripes Black Shorts				

My first trophy came when I won a penalty competition at Millwall FC when I was 13. I even had my picture in their programme.

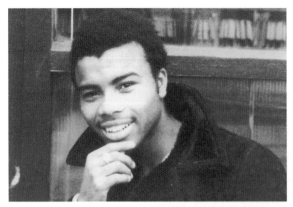

Trying to look cool in my sheepskin coat, the same one I wore for my post-match interview with John Motson after my debut at Old Trafford.

Proudly posing for a picture in my Southampton away kit. I sent this to Jenny during my first year at the club.

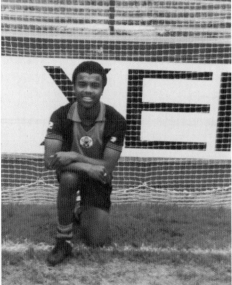

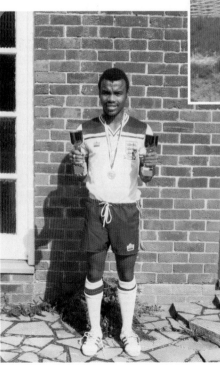

My first step on the international ladder. I'm showing off some of the trophies I won for the England youth team as a 17 year old.

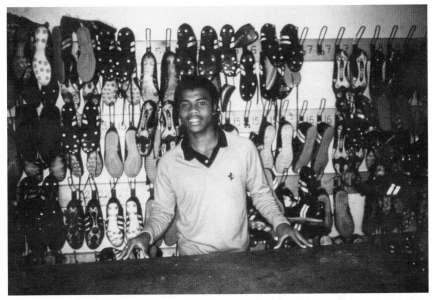

I may have played in the Southampton first team at 16, but that didn't mean I got out of all the apprentices' chores. Here I am in the boot room at The Dell.

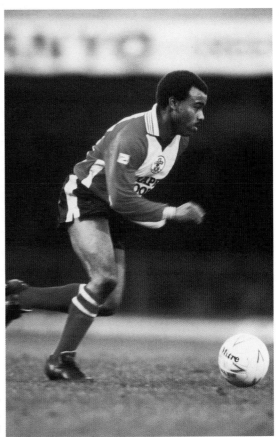

Doing what I did best, running with the ball at my feet.
© Getty Images

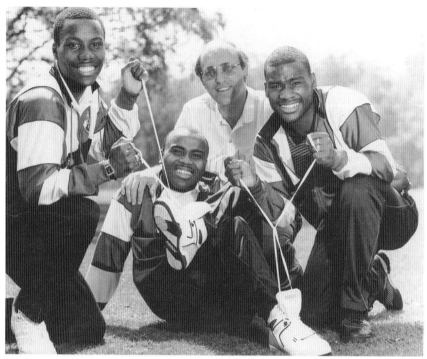

With my brothers, Rodney (left) and Raymond (right) along with Bob Higgins in our Southampton days.

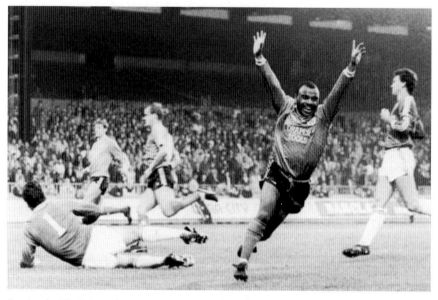

Scoring for The Saints always gave me a thrill. © Empics

Jenny and I caused a bit of a stir at one of the Manchester United Christmas parties when we turned up dressed as a KKK member and a slave.

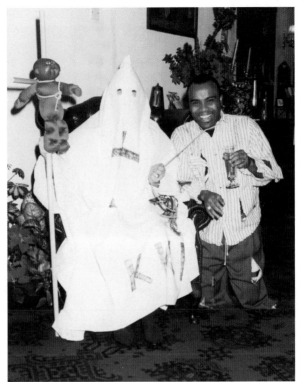

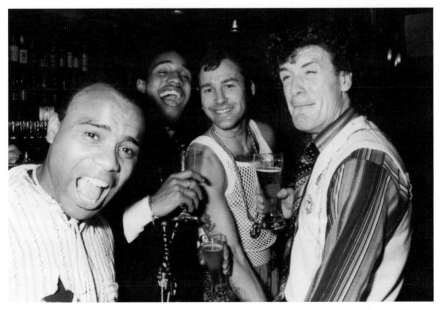

Getting into the festive spirit at the same party, along with Paul Ince, Bryan Robson and Mark Hughes.

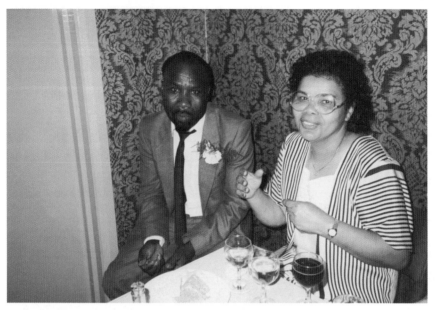

Mum and dad.

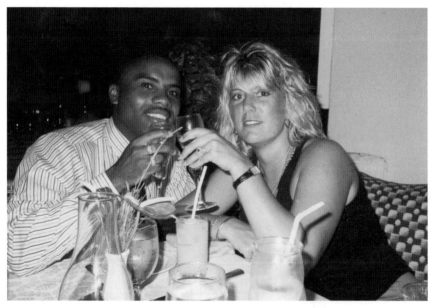

On honeymoon with Jenny in 1988.

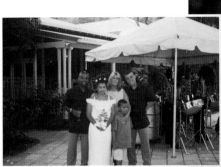

A family shot taken at Rodney's wedding in 2000. Jenny and me with Elisha, Thaila and Remi.

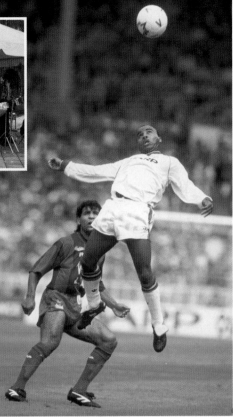

Making the most of my height (!) in the FA Cup final.
© *Getty Images*

Still celebrating the Cup Final win. Here I am with boxer Nigel Benn at Paul Ince's wedding.

Jenny, Elisha and me with the Cup that helped me fulfil a dream.

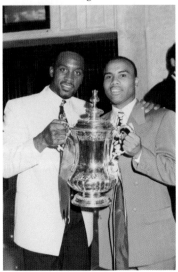

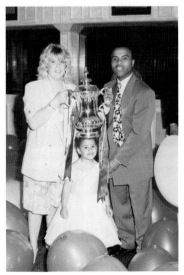

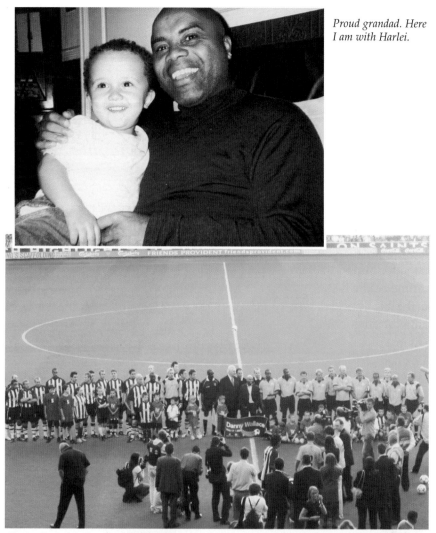

Proud grandad. Here I am with Harlei.

Above: One of the best nights of my life. My testimonial at Southampton in 2004.

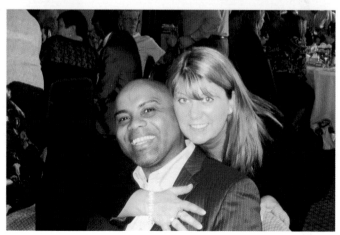

Jen and me in 2005.

one of the new kids in Fergie's family. There were others who were just as talented a bit further down the line, the likes of David Beckham, Gary Neville, Paul Scholes and Nicky Butt. A new era in domestic football was about to emerge, and I feared I would be in no fit state to compete for a place in it.

It was during the summer that I got my clearest indication yet that my days as a United player were numbered. If the start of the previous season had got off on a sour note when I injured my groin against Liverpool at Wembley, the news I got twelve months later was hardly likely to boost my low self-confidence. Alan Shearer had made a name for himself at Southampton and it seemed to be only a matter of time before he left the club. Just as everyone was looking forward to the big kick-off there were stories in all the newspapers about United trying to prise him away from Southampton using me as the bait in a proposed two-way deal. It seemed pretty obvious to me that Alex had given up on me. I suppose that if I was in his shoes I might have done the same. I don't ever think he believed I was putting it on, because he could see how desperate I was to get back into the first team whenever I was out injured, but at the same time he'd probably come to the conclusion that he'd bought an injury-prone player.

My brother Rodney's situation was similar to Shearer's. While my career seemed to be going backwards, his had gone into overdrive. He'd emerged as one of the best young players around and had started to think that he should move away and join a bigger club. The fact that it had all gone belly-up for me didn't seem to put Rod off, and I think he decided that he wasn't going to sign a new contract with the club; instead, he would let his current deal run out, allowing other clubs who might be interested to come in for him. Ray hadn't fared quite so well, and although he was in the Southampton first-team squad he'd found it difficult to pin down a regular spot and had to be content to play much of his football in the reserves. I could certainly sympathise with him. I knew all about reserve matches. In fact, I was becoming an expert in them, and later on I actually became the reserve-team captain at United. Not bad for a £1.2 million player who was supposed to take Old Trafford by storm!

During that summer of 1991 Rodney got the big move he was hoping for. The Leeds manager, Howard Wilkinson, decided to take Raymond too as part of a package that priced Rod at £1.6 million and Ray at £100,000. Suddenly, all three of us were getting a taste of life in the north.

The Shearer stories stayed around for a while, and the new Southampton manager, Ian Branfoot, was apparently keen to get me back at The Dell. Nothing more came of it, though, which meant I just had to put it all down to paper talk and get on with the business of trying to earn a place in the United team. But on that front things just seemed to go from bad to worse. The injuries were as frequent as ever, and I think I got to the stage where I was going out on to the pitch almost expecting the worst to happen. As a consequence, by the end of the year I was struggling. Fergie had spent too long waiting for me to deliver the goods, and in December 1991 he drew a line and put me on the transfer list.

CHAPTER TEN

PARTING SHOTS

The meeting I had with Alex Ferguson was pleasant enough, and I think we both came out of it thinking that my going on the list was the right thing to do. It would be a chance for me to start afresh with a new club, and from United's point of view it gave them the opportunity to cut their losses. Alex knew he wasn't going to get the same sort of money he'd paid for me, but they had to try to obtain something.

It wasn't exactly the best Christmas present I could have had that December, but I hoped that a club would come in during the New Year and give me the opportunity to put the disappointment of my time with United behind me. The move just hadn't worked out, but at least I had no doubt in my own mind that without all those injuries I would have made a success of my time at Old Trafford. Despite all my problems I really liked the club, and when I was fit I used to love going to The Cliff; maybe I appreciated it more than most because of all those times when I had to sit out sessions. As strange as it may sound, I never got to the point where I thought there might be something more serious wrong with me. As far as I was concerned it was just a crop of unfortunate injuries. It wasn't just one recurring type of injury, and because of that I don't think the club's medical staff had any suspicions about an underlying condition. I still had confidence in my own ability and just wanted to prove I could play. Although things hadn't gone well for me at United I knew others thought I had ability. I was picked for some England B internationals, which was a nice confidence boost. I think the fact that Lawrie McMenemy was by this time assistant to the new

England manager, Graham Taylor, certainly had a bearing on me being selected, but it was the sort of thing that gave me hope of being able to change my situation.

As soon as my place on the transfer list became public there were more stories linking me with a return to The Dell in part-exchange for Alan Shearer. Alan's reputation had continued to grow, and the idea of United signing one of the brightest young strikers in the game must have been appealing to Alex at a time when he had a side which was beginning to win trophies and was looking to challenge for the league title. As for me, I just hoped I could get a move. Apart from Southampton, I was also linked with West Ham, which would certainly have suited me. Bob Higgins was hoping that Billy Bonds, who was the Hammers' manager at the time, would show some interest, but we heard nothing. There was also talk of Kenny Dalglish thinking about making a bid as he tried to get Blackburn promoted from the Second Division, backed by the financial muscle of Jack Walker. Once again there was a lot of speculation, and once again no official bid.

Ironically, virtually from the day I was put on the list I stayed injury free and began to look good in the reserves, knocking in goals and generally playing well. The fact that I was fit and relaxed probably helped and I actually enjoyed the games, even if some of them were played in front of only a handful of people. I think it was my form in the reserves that prompted all the talk about a move to Blackburn in the first place, and I knew that on a few occasions there were people from other clubs checking on my form and fitness. I did get some games in the first team in 1991/92, but I certainly wasn't first choice and hadn't played in a league match since May 1991. As an indication of how far I'd slipped down the ladder, when United got to the Rumbelows Cup final for the second year running, I again had to make do with a seat in the stands. I'd gone from playing in two FA Cup final matches to being no more than a spectator in the Wembley stands. By the early summer of 1992 I'd reached the stage where I was actually embarrassed by the way things had turned out for me. I knew it was nobody's fault, but in many ways that only seemed to make it worse. It would have been nice to be able to point the finger at someone and say that because of them I had been left out in the cold, but that simply wasn't the case.

It's often said that football is a funny old game, and there's no doubt that one of the qualities you have to have as a player is resilience. You get all sorts of ups and downs and you have to accept them and bounce back in the best way you can. The one thing you have to do is take any chances that come your way, so whenever I found myself back in the side I wanted to make sure I enjoyed every minute of it. The team were flying that season, so at least when I did play I was part of a side that was full of confidence and pressing hard for the league title, even if I did only have a bit part to play.

One of the other teams trying to win the championship was Leeds, and someone who certainly didn't have a bit part with them was my brother Rodney. He had really blossomed at Elland Road and was one of the big factors in them doing so well in what was to be the last season before the Premiership was formed. In the end it was Howard Wilkinson's boys who came out on top, winning the title by four points from us. I was really pleased for Rodney and for Raymond, although he hadn't really been involved to any great extent. I knew how much it meant to get off to a good start with a new club, and to pick up a league championship medal in your first season was a brilliant way to begin your career. Raymond had actually started lodging with us by this stage, so Jenny was back in the familiar old routine, although she only had two of the Wallace boys to look after this time, because Rod decided to stay in a flat in Leeds.

As the season came to a close I found myself in a bit of a football limbo. I knew I wasn't an automatic choice with United – in fact I was struggling even to get a look-in – and at the same time nobody seemed interested in taking me, because there were no bids from other clubs. I was back in the situation of having to prepare for a new season knowing that I was unlikely to play too much of a part in it. But I'm an optimist. I knew that things would change, so once again I was determined to get myself as fit as possible so that I was in with a chance to turn things around.

Unfortunately, when it came to trying to prove that I still had a future with United I managed to do a good job of shooting myself in the foot during a pre-season tour in Sweden. Like most clubs when they are on tour, the manager decides what time he wants his players in their rooms at night. Going to Sweden might sound nice enough, but the real purpose of the trip was for us to train and get some matches under our belts against the local opposition. The curfew was set at ten p.m., but Paul Ince, Clayton Blackmore and I decided one night that the deadline was a bit early and we fancied sampling some of the nightlife, so we wandered down to a nightclub in the hotel for a few drinks and a bit of fun. The evening soon got out of hand and ended with a fire-extinguisher being set off. The manager of the hotel wasn't best pleased when he heard about what had happened and immediately let Fergie know what three of his players had been up to. Needless to say, Alex wasn't too pleased either.

When we got back to Manchester I had to go and see him. My excuse that because it was a pre-season tour we thought there wasn't any real curfew didn't really go down too well. Things got a bit heated in his office, with him having a go at me and letting me know exactly how he felt about what I'd done. I realise now that it was a stupid thing to have got involved in, and maybe part of the reason for doing it was because I was so fed up with my situation at the club. Having a couple of drinks and a bit of a laugh with my mates just seemed like innocent fun. I didn't say that to Fergie though, so maybe he thought I just couldn't be bothered any more after all the set-backs I'd had. There was no way I was going to come out of it looking good, and just to emphasise the fact that there was only ever one winner in a situation like that, he fined me two weeks' wages, making it one of the most expensive nights out I'd ever had in my life.

Nobody tended to get the better of Fergie. It was always clear who was the boss around the place, although that didn't stop a few of the lads having a go back. There was one incident while I was with United that left even Alex lost for words. He was unhappy with Incy after one game and had a bit of a blast at him. Paul was hardly a shrinking violet, and with a nickname like 'The Guvnor' he wasn't about to take a ticking-off lying down. In fact, Incy usually puffed out his chest and stood toe to toe with Alex if the two of them were having a go at each other. On this particular occasion Paul was really pissed off with Fergie, and a couple of days later when we all arrived for training he was still steaming at what had gone on. 'I ain't having it, Dan,' he told me as we all got out of our cars. 'What he said was out of order. Let's see what he has to say when he sees this.' And then, with the biggest grin you've ever seen, he went to the boot of his car and pulled out a gun. Actually it was an air rifle, but it was still a mean-looking thing and I wouldn't have wanted to be on the wrong end of it.

Incy took the gun and ran up the stairs to Alex's office. The door was slightly open, so Paul gave it a little nudge to open it even more before slowly poking the end of the barrel into the room. Suddenly there was a loud bang, and then a shout from inside the office. Heaven knows what Fergie thought or did when he saw the gun and then heard the shot, but Incy didn't wait to find out: he raced back down the stairs leaving a wide-eyed and red-faced Fergie swearing at the entrance to his office. I think only Alex and his underpants knew the extent of the shock he'd been given by the stunt, but once he'd got over the surprise he took it well and there were a lot of laughs all round.

I think Alex actually liked having strong characters and personalities in his team. He was confident enough in his own man-management skills to take some players on who other people might have steered clear of. He never treated you like a kid, but at the same time expected a player to behave in a certain way and not do stupid things. He had a word with me a couple of times because people had phoned the club and said they'd seen me out drinking in the middle of the week. It was nothing heavy – I was probably only having a couple of beers – but Alex was aware of the effect it could have with the supporters and on the club. He liked discipline, but he was sensible about what he asked of his players. It's well known that there were some heavy drinkers at the club before I went there, and when I was with United Bryan Robson was hardly a choirboy when it came to alcohol, but he was also a fantastic player who was the heartbeat of the side. I think Fergie allowed him a certain amount of freedom to go out and enjoy himself, because he knew that Robbo would always turn up for training and be ready to lead from the front. He was a real leader on and off the pitch, and his wife, Denise, was really nice to all the other players' wives and girlfriends.

I have to say that although things didn't go as well as they might have done for me on the pitch, I got on really well with all the players. As I said, we didn't socialise with them that much, but that was due to location as much as anything else: we lived on the north side of Manchester and lots of them lived to the south, in places like Knutsford and Wilmslow. Incy was the exception when it came to socialising. We seemed to hit it off right away, and Jenny got on well with Claire, his girlfriend at the time, who later went on to become his wife. When we were staying at the Ramada in the early months, Paul, Gary Pallister and I used to take turns each morning to drive into training, and in the afternoons I would often spend quite a bit of time with Incy in the betting shop. We both liked to have a flutter, and with time on our hands it was easy to just wander down to the bookies to indulge our hobby.

Incy was the life and soul of any social event, but even he was left open-mouthed one Christmas at the annual players' party. It was a fancy dress theme, and he probably thought he looked good dressed as a vicar – that was until Jen and I walked in and the place was almost stunned into silence. Jenny was dressed in a Ku Klux Klan outfit and I was dressed as a slave. Worse still, she had me on a chain with a collar round my neck. I think a few people were a bit surprised and didn't know how to react, but we liked it. It appealed to our sense of humour, which always was a bit on the sick side. Paul was also the practical joker of the squad, and he was often helped by Ryan Giggs. If someone had had a practical joke played on them, the first place to look for the culprits would be Incy and Giggsy. A lot of the time it wasn't very sophisticated stuff, just things like players having the tops of their socks cut off, or pins put in their underpants. It was childish, I know, but enough to get a bunch of overgrown kids who play football for a living laughing after a training session on a cold winter's day.

I've already mentioned that Ryan began to emerge in 1991/92 as a real talent in the team, and soon after the 1992/93 season got underway the Old Trafford faithful also saw the likes of Beckham, Neville and Butt make the step-up to first-team level, although it was later on in their careers with the club that they really started to make an impact. Big Dion Dublin also joined United in the summer of 1992 from Cambridge for more than £1 million, and I suppose that in comparison with what happened to him shortly after coming to the club I must have looked lucky. Poor Dion broke his leg and damaged ligaments in his third game for United and ended up making only a handful of starts in the two years he was with the club.

There was also another new arrival at Old Trafford towards the end of the year, and he was to have a huge influence on the team and the club during the time he spent in Manchester. Eric Cantona had just helped Leeds win the league title, and when he joined in November I got to see at first hand just what a good player he was. I'd already heard from my brothers that the Frenchman was a bit special, and from the moment he set foot in Old Trafford he seemed to lift the team with his skill and ability, taking United to the next level and making them a genuine force in the first season of the Premier League. Eric was a tremendous trainer and a great professional. He would be out there practising with the ball before training started and after it finished. He seemed to shun all the usual trappings of a successful footballer and was quite happy to live in a modest house. He loved his football and got on well with the players. I think they could see what a big talent he was, and it was no coincidence that the team really seemed to click once he had arrived at the club.

After that late-night incident in Sweden, I really buckled down to training and got myself fit. I was determined to give it the best shot I had. Even if United didn't want me I hoped that my performances in the reserves might get me a move and give me the new start I wanted.

I'd heard that Alex was ready to sell me for around £600,000, but there hadn't been any takers. I decided it was up to me to make people sit up and take notice. I finally got a high-profile chance on 23 September in a Coca-Cola (League) Cup tie at Brighton. The team had a poor game but I played well and scored our goal in the 1–1 draw. Not only did I grab the headlines, I also got praise from Alex after the match; he admitted that my performance had opened the door again for me in the first team. It was like music to my ears, and for a month or two it really did seem as though it could be a turning point for me. But my hopes were again short-lived, and while United marched on in the Premiership, eventually claiming their first championship title since 1967, I spent most of the next five months or so either in the reserves or on the treatment table, which left me feeling unhappy, frustrated and desperate to end my Old Trafford nightmare.

It was probably a build-up of those feelings that led to me having a go at Alex. I'd had a couple of run-ins with him during my time at the club, but they were really nothing to get upset about. Once, he bollocked me for something or other and in the process let me know he felt let down by the way I'd played by shouting, 'To think I even put you in the squad for the Cup Winners' Cup final instead of my own son!' But that outburst was nothing compared to what happened at half-time during one reserve game early in 1993. I'd been having real trouble getting going in the match; in fact, I just couldn't run. It wasn't that I was unfit, it was simply that my legs felt heavy and I had no real zip to my game. I knew I wasn't playing well, so I didn't need Fergie coming into the dressing room to tell me.

'You're an absolute disgrace,' he said, not really expecting a reply.

To be honest, in normal circumstances he wouldn't have got one. But I'd just about had enough. I knew I was trying my hardest out on the pitch, it's just that physically I wasn't able to do what I wanted to do.

'Why don't you fuck off and leave me alone!' I shouted, and as the words came out of my mouth I could see Alex's face starting to turn red.

'Right, you,' he said, pointing his finger at me. 'Get your kit off and fuck off out of here.' With that, he turned around and walked out, leaving me sitting in the dressing room fuming.

I threw my shirt down in front of me and kicked it along the floor. I was angry and frustrated. On top of that I'd just told the manager to fuck off. Not the best night of my career. I got showered and stormed out of the ground, arriving home before the match had even finished. I was in a foul mood all night, but by the time I woke up the next morning the fury had lifted and I began to regret what I had done. I drove to the training ground and as soon as I saw Alex I asked if I could talk to him in his office. I apologised for what I'd done the night before and told him it was completely out of character for me, which I think he probably knew was true. I'd always had respect for the managers and coaches I'd worked with, and I told Fergie that I had been out of order to swear at him. He listened to me and said he understood that I was frustrated and not to think any more about it. I came out feeling that the matter was closed. I was also pleased that I had a manager who was big enough to handle something like that in the way he had done.

I'm sure it was pure coincidence, but it wasn't too long after that meeting that I was told Millwall had been on to the club enquiring about me, and United had agreed that they could have me on a three-month loan if I was happy to go. It was a chance for me to get a run of games, and even though Millwall were in the First Division I knew they probably offered me the best opportunity I would get to show that I could still play. They were also my local club, as I'd lived only minutes away from their ground when I was a kid in Deptford. I had a lot of family and friends down in that part of London and the more I thought about it the more the loan began to appeal to me.

I decided to give it a go, so in March, as United continued to move away from their nearest rivals in the battle for the first ever Premiership title, I headed south to try to recapture the sort of form I still thought I was capable of.

CHAPTER ELEVEN

GETTING THE BLUES

Millwall fans might not have the best of reputations in football, and there's no doubt that over the years the club has had its fair share of bad publicity, but it also happens to be one of the friendliest clubs you could wish to play for. I knew that the trick to success would be winning the fans over straight away, and if that happened they would give me great support. They loved players who put everything into their game when they pulled on the Millwall shirt, and I knew that if I stayed fit and was picked, I could do a job for them. Dropping down a division for a few months didn't bother me, even though it was the first time in my career that I'd played outside the top flight. I just wanted the chance to play regular first-team football again, and Mick McCarthy, who was the Millwall manager at the time, was prepared to give me that opportunity. And I was happy to go there because The Den held happy memories for me: as an eleven-year-old I won a half-time penalty competition there and was presented with the first football trophy I ever won. It was also quite an exciting time for the club when I joined because when the season ended they were due to move from their ground into a brand-new stadium about a mile down the road.

Once the deal had been agreed I moved south to stay with my mum and dad in Deptford during the week and then travelled back to Jenny and the family home at weekends. Millwall trained at New Eltham, which was just a short drive from my parents' place, and I started to look forward to the three months I would have back home.

Mick was a nice guy and he outlined what he wanted from me and how he thought the team would benefit from my pace and experience, but I can't honestly say that either he or the Millwall faithful got much of a chance to enjoy anything I did, and the only lasting impression I left with them was of a player who hardly managed to play. Once again I found myself having most of my conversations with the manager from the treatment table, and once again the injuries weren't serious, but they did mean that during the entire time I was back in London with Millwall I was never fit enough to play regularly. Poor Mick couldn't have been nicer about it, but he must have felt upset at getting someone like me in to do a job and then finding that he wasn't able to use me for long periods. So what I'd hoped would be the perfect place to get some games and show people I was back to my best turned out to be another frustrating chapter in what was becoming the story of my footballing decline.

During my time in London, United romped away with the Premier League title, finishing the season ten points ahead of Aston Villa in second place. It was a great achievement for Alex and the lads, and of course I was delighted for them, but in some ways winning the title seemed to make me feel more sidelined than ever. I would have loved to be part of that championship-winning side, but the truth was that I'd slipped way down the ladder. United as a club had moved on, and at the same time Danny Wallace the player had moved backwards. As I packed my bags and prepared to travel north at the season's end, it was difficult to know what to do next.

The optimist in me kept saying that things would be all right, that there was no way the injuries could continue to crop up in the way they had done. But I also knew that I'd now been saying the same thing for the last few years, and I was the sort of player who needed to play regularly. The more I played the better I got, or at least that was the way it had been during my time at Southampton. I was 29 years old. I should have been at the peak of my career, but things had gone badly off the rails for me and I was beginning to have a tough time, not just physically but also mentally.

Around this time Jenny began to see a change in me at home as well. Although I've never been an extrovert I've always been confident as a footballer and playing the game for a living always made me happy. Jen and I had our ups and downs like any other couple, and I'd be the first to admit that I hadn't always treated her the way I should have, but nobody knew me better than she did and nobody could understand me better as a person. She could see how upset I was getting with the way my football career was going, and she's since told me that she noticed my confidence beginning to drain away at that time. It was no surprise really, because after that brief spell at Millwall, and because of the way it ended, I really couldn't see a way out. The only good thing about it all was that financially I was doing all right. I was still under my original contract at United and it had another year to run. At the beginning of July 1993 I was due to get a six-figure basic for the first time in my life, because my salary had gone up each year since signing for the club and at that time I was on £100,000 a year. The money was nice, but the football meant more. Jenny and I have never been overly materialistic. It was always good to know that I was earning a more than decent wage, but we weren't extravagant in the way we lived our lives and we certainly didn't go in for things like big houses and flash cars. I knew that if I was going to go to another club I would have to take a drop in wages, but that didn't matter. The main thing was actually finding a club that would be willing to take a gamble on me.

There was pretty strong interest from the French club Le Havre, and I seriously considered the prospect. I thought that maybe I could go over there each week and then come back after matches, because there was no way we were going to just sell up and go over there as a family. But on reflection I thought it would be too much of an upheaval for Jen and the kids and decided instead to stay and see what else might happen.

After their initial interest about eighteen months earlier when I had first gone on the transfer list, I'd heard nothing more about Southampton wanting to take me back to The Dell. But Ian Branfoot, who had been at the club as youth-team coach during the time I was there, was still the manager and obviously thought I could do a job despite the problems I'd had at United because he got in touch and asked about the possibility of signing me. The new season had just started, it was clear that I wasn't going to get a look-in at United, and Alex Ferguson agreed that I could go down and talk to them, believing that it was probably the sort of move that would suit me. But the truth was that although I knew I had to get away from United, I didn't really feel Southampton offered the sort of fresh start I needed.

Don't get me wrong, when I played for Southampton I absolutely loved the club and the fans, and still do to this day, but I had a gut feeling that going back to the club I had left was not a good move. Once you make a break like that in football I think it's better to stick with it. If you go back, comparisons will always be made; people will look back and remember the way you were. I had great times at The Dell, and I have some great memories. I didn't want to spoil that and put added pressure on myself by going to a club where so many people already knew me. But at the same time I was realistic enough to know that there wasn't exactly a line of clubs waiting to sign me, so I decided to go down and at least talk about a move.

Bob Higgins was no longer looking after me as my agent. He had always really been more of a friend than an agent anyway. When my contract with him ran out I decided not to sign another agreement. Bob wasn't upset by it and we stayed in contact, but with him living in the south and me in the north there didn't really seem to be the need for us to carry on with the business arrangement we'd previously had. Instead, I went down for the meeting accompanied by Ambrose Mendy, who had acted for Paul Ince in the past and had also made a name for himself in boxing, looking after the likes of Nigel Benn. We spoke with Branfoot for about an hour, and it was clear he wanted me to sign. The money on offer was about half what I was earning at United, but I'd expected that. The main problem was that all through the meeting I had this feeling that it wouldn't be the right move for me. By the time I got to Manchester my mind was made up: again, I'd sit it out and hope that another club came along, or a miracle happened and I got the chance to play for United once more.

The next day I turned up for training. 'What the fuck are you doing here?' Fergie asked when he saw me. 'I thought you'd gone.' It was said with a smile, but it was clear that he hadn't expected me back from Southampton. It was another obvious indication to me that I was very much surplus to requirements at Old Trafford. United had a very different team and a very different squad. They were the Premier League champions, and you could tell they were only going to get better. It would have been lovely to be a part of all that, but my time there was over. All I could hope for was for another club to put me out of my misery, otherwise I knew I was in for a slow, lingering career death in the reserves.

Not long after the offer from Southampton another came in, this time from Birmingham City. They were a big club in a big city, and when I went along there I immediately liked their manager Terry Cooper, who had been a great full-back with Leeds and England. I was under the impression that United would let me go on a free transfer. It made sense because they wanted to get rid of me, and if they had to write off all the £1.2 million they'd paid for me, at least they would be saving money on my wages for the final year of my contract, and it made me more attractive to any possible buying club. But as I sat with Birmingham's managing director, Karren Brady, it soon became apparent that United wanted a fee. In fact, they wanted £250,000. I remember sitting in her office while she was on the phone to Alex and hearing her ask exactly how much he wanted for me. I'd hoped that a free transfer might help me negotiate a bit more on my contract, but it wasn't to be, and in the end I was just happy to get a deal sorted out, even if it did mean a drop of about £800 per week.

Once I'd put pen to paper I felt a sense of relief. Signing for United had been one of the biggest thrills of my life, and winning the FA Cup was magnificent, but in the three years that had followed it had all gone badly wrong for me. I'd had so many false dawns during those years when I thought I was over the worst times, before finding out that just wasn't the case. Birmingham offered me new hope. I was fit when I signed in October 1993 and raring to go. I wanted to let the Blues fans see they had bought a player who would give everything he had for the team and entertain them at the same time.

When I turned up for training on my first day all my old enthusiasm was there and I really enjoyed myself. Terry Cooper gave a lot of encouragement to his team and I think the players liked him. As a player, although he was a full-back, he was known for the way he made surging runs down the wing, and I got the impression that he loved the thought of me doing the same for his team. I was looking forward to working with him, but sadly our association was short-lived. Just a few weeks after my arrival Terry was sacked and Barry Fry moved in as the new manager. I knew nothing about Fry other than the fact that he always came across as a larger than life charac-ter, but after working with him for a few days I'd made my mind up – I simply didn't like the man or his methods.

Actually, to say he had a method would be overstating things a bit as far as I'm concerned. Fry seemed to revel in working in a chaotic atmosphere, and it appeared to me that he was the one who created the chaos. As soon as he arrived there were players coming and going on the transfer market, so much so that you didn't really know who people were at times. The training wasn't great either, and I soon realised he was very different to the managers I'd been used to. I had a lot of respect for Lawrie, Fergie and Chris Nicholl, but I found it very difficult to take to Barry Fry. He didn't seem to have any of the man-management skills that had been such a big part of the way the other three went about their business. You never really knew what to expect with Fry. One minute he'd be trying to make jokes, the next he'd be barking out instructions as if he was talking to a bunch of schoolboys. The snide comments he would make later on during my time at the club really got to me. I suppose his style and methods might have appealed to some players, but they certainly weren't what I was looking for when I joined the club. The simple fact was that I didn't have much of a choice. Birmingham had given me a chance to kick-start my career and I was grateful for the opportunity, although I have to say that had Fry been in charge when they came in for me I would never have signed for them. Mind you, I'm not sure he would have gone for me if he had been the boss.

Just to make things worse, I only played a couple of games in the first team before getting injured. It was back to the treatment room once again for me, and in the eighteen months I spent at St Andrews that became a depressingly familiar story for me. They seemed to occur with even greater frequency than they had done at United, and what I had hoped would be a new start for me quickly became another one of those false dawns. It was apparent very quickly that I was back to square one.

I used to travel every day from our house in Worsley to the Birmingham training ground, which was a journey of about 80 minutes. Quite often during the trip I would wonder just what I'd got myself into. The fact that I was on the treatment table for long periods didn't endear me to Fry. I often heard him making comments; perhaps he didn't believe I was genuinely out of action all the time. To be fair to him, it must have seemed strange that I was picking up so many injuries, and certainly I was no use out of the team, particularly as Birmingham were struggling in the First Division at the time. But the truth was that not only was I picking up injuries with greater frequency, my body was beginning to feel strange as well. I didn't tell anyone, and in my own mind I think I put it down to natural wear and tear, but I knew the aches and pains I had now were different to anything I'd experienced before. In the past I would get an injury, have some treatment and be out of action for a while, but when I was able to start training again my body felt normal. It was then just a case of building up my fitness levels before playing football again, which was usually in a reserve match. At Birmingham, the same sort of injuries were taking me longer to recover from, and when they cleared up I found it much harder to get back to a level of fitness I felt happy with. Quite often my legs would feel heavy and I would be aching after a training session, when in the past I would have done the same amount of work and thought nothing of it. I felt myself struggling throughout that first season with Birmingham, and on the pitch the team was struggling as well. All of Fry's wheeling and dealing couldn't prevent the club from being relegated in May 1994 to life in the Second Division.

If things hadn't worked out too well for me during that first season I at least had the pleasure of becoming a dad again during the summer, when Jenny gave birth to a second boy, who we named

Thaila. It was great to have a new baby and we were both thrilled when he arrived right at the beginning of the new season. In fact, I just about had time to see him being born before dashing off to play in a game.

I wasn't sure what to expect of life in the Second Division. Obviously the standard of football wasn't going to be as good as I'd been used to in the past, but that didn't really worry me at the time; all that concerned me was actually playing in the first team. Football was football as far as I was concerned, and kicking a ball around was all I ever wanted to do. Not being able to do that was horrible, and the one thing all the injuries had done was to make me more aware than ever how lucky I was to be a footballer and to make me want to play for as long as I could. As far as I was concerned I'd missed the chance to make the most of things in recent years and I was determined to make up for that.

When I returned for pre-season training I wanted to let Barry Fry know that I was ready to play my part in trying to bounce the club straight back into the First Division. Part of the training one day involved a road run, something that had never been a problem to me in the past. Fry wasn't the sort of manager to get too involved in general training and coaching throughout the week – he left that to his coaches – but when it came to pre-season he did put in an appearance. During the course of the road run I suddenly became aware that I was struggling. I wasn't gasping for breath, and I didn't feel as though I wasn't fit enough. Instead it was another kind of pain which really began to unnerve me. I felt as if I had a rod in my back, and I couldn't move freely. Fry caught sight of me, and in his usual way shouted some comment about me having to make sure I kept up with the rest, but as he said the words my mind was somewhere else. He might have been trying to take the piss or to have a go at me, but I didn't really care. What I did care about was the horrible feeling I had in my back. It wasn't a spasm, just a stiffness and a sharp ache which really worried me. I didn't want to let anyone know about it and tried to carry on as best I could, but it was a horrible feeling. I'd never experienced anything like it before.

I managed to get through the pre-season training without any more problems with my back, and after the birth of Thaila everything seemed to be settling down nicely. But I should have known it wouldn't last. Within five months Jenny's joy at having a new baby was shattered when she had a miscarriage. We obviously hadn't planned to have another baby so quickly, but Jenny did become pregnant again and it was a horrific experience for her to lose the baby in January 1995. Once again I hadn't been having the best of times on the playing front, and I don't suppose I was too much fun to live with at the time. I'd arranged for some friends and their kids to come up on the weekend after my birthday to help me celebrate being 31 years old, and I suppose I also thought it might help cheer me up a bit. All the arrangements had been made a few weeks earlier and I was looking forward to it, but then Jenny miscarried and had to go into hospital overnight. She was naturally in a bit of a state when she got back home the next day and asked me to cancel the weekend, but I didn't bother.

I find it hard to believe now that I acted the way I did. My wife had just lost a baby, emotionally she was on the floor, but instead of thinking about how she felt I went ahead and did what I wanted to do almost as if she didn't exist. I might have been having problems with my playing career, but they were nothing compared to what poor Jen was experiencing at the time. It was probably one of the most selfish things I've ever done in my life, and something I will always regret. It wasn't just a case of me not thinking straight, it was a case of me not thinking at all. Jenny had been with me for so long I'd started to take her for granted. I was self-centred enough to do something like arrange a night out with my mates at a time when my wife had just lost one baby and was still caring for another. And just to add to her misery, some of our friends brought their own kids with them that weekend, which made Jenny feel even more of a wreck. I was completely oblivious to it all, or at least I was too wrapped up in my own world to worry about anyone else.

I went out on the town leaving Jenny at home, but it wasn't too long before I got a call while I was in a club and heard Jenny screaming down the other end of the phone threatening to walk out not only on me but also the baby. Thankfully the call brought me to my senses and I realised what a complete bastard I'd been. I raced home with tears streaming down my face and rushed into the bedroom. I could see that Jenny had gone berserk and smashed the room to pieces. She was screaming at me and crying as well. We both sat on the bed sobbing, emotionally drained and unable to speak. I think we were both at different stages of depression, and we were dealing with it in different ways. The trouble was we were doing it separately rather than together. Instead of talking to each other we'd been bottling up our feelings.

The fact that I went ahead with going out that night brought things to a head. I was beginning to resent my life, feeling hard done by because of what was happening with my football career; it seemed as though everything was going against me. As far as I was concerned it was all about me and nobody else, not even my wife and family. I might have had it bad, but now, when I thought of what poor Jenny had dealt with in the previous few months, it filled me with guilt. Not only had she given birth and had a miscarriage, she was also the one who'd had most to do in terms of helping our daughter cope with the news that she was a diabetic. Little Elisha was only eight years old but had started to lose weight and clearly wasn't well. Jenny helped her come to terms with the news that she would have to start injecting herself with insulin every day for the rest of her life. On top of that she was looking after Remi, and then she had to face a husband who probably came home looking as though he had the weight of the world on his shoulders. No wonder she cracked up that night.

It was clear Jenny wasn't well, and although the bedroom was in a mess after the way she'd bashed it about, she refused to come out. I thought it best to stick around, so I phoned the club and explained the situation, telling them that I was going to take some time off to look after my wife. I was left in no doubt that I would be in big trouble if I didn't show up for training. I couldn't believe it. My wife had just had a miscarriage, she was now in the middle of what appeared to be a nervous breakdown, and they were basically telling me to get my arse into training or face the consequences. I tried to explain to Jenny that I had to go in and that I'd be straight back after training. She was still upset and very emotional, but we at least started to talk to each other and she was calm enough to agree that I should go in.

I drove to training in a terrible mood because of what they had made me do. I just couldn't accept that a football club should be any different to another business. Had I been working in an office or a factory I'm sure my employers would have given me compassionate leave to be with my wife after what had happened, but that didn't seem to apply to Birmingham. Still, I decided not to go in and have a row. Instead, I just kept my head down and got on with what I was asked to do without really saying anything to the manager or the coaching staff, though the situation certainly didn't help my personal relationship with Barry Fry. As far as I was concerned he was the manager, so he presumably made the decisions about whether or not a player should be allowed to miss training.

Talking to Jenny during that miserable period in our lives helped both of us in many ways. I think we said a lot of things that needed saying, and we gradually started to communicate properly again. Jenny initially remained reluctant to come out of the bedroom, and I think she stayed in there for about five days before emerging. The key to her coming out was our daughter. She might have been only eight years old, but she had seen and heard what had been going on and was aware that the little brother or sister she thought she might be getting had died. Jenny later told me that Elisha had taken a drink in for her one morning and had told her, 'It's not just you that's lost the baby, Mum.' It had a profound effect on Jenny and she realised that, as upsetting as the whole experience had been, she still had her children and family who were there for her. It was a very emotional time for everyone, one of the worst weeks of our lives, but I'm convinced the relationship between Jenny and me was stronger afterwards, and I'm sure it helped us prepare as a couple for what was to come along a couple of years later.

It was clear that things were not working out for me at St Andrews, and once again I was into the familiar cycle of injuries, physio, and then a reserve game. It had almost become second nature to me, and now getting any kind of match under my belt was a bonus. I hadn't been feeling right since that day in pre-season when my back really began to hurt on the road run. I'd muddled through, but my body wasn't holding up in the way it had done in the past. I thought that perhaps because I'd been playing in the professional game since I was sixteen I was now, fifteen years later, beginning to suffer some side-effects. I didn't feel as lively as I usually did and training for two hours was making me weary. I'd got used to having to deal with the physical effects of being injured on many occasions, but suddenly there was a whole new mental side to it all as well. I started to worry about what was happening and was also much more aware of my physical movements, which meant that I wasn't doing the sort of things with the ball that had always come naturally to me. It all came to a head during a reserve game when I had an experience that I found both frightening and shocking.

Like lots of other football-mad kids, when I was a youngster living at home with my parents I would sometimes have a balloon in the house which I would use as a football. It was great, because you could belt the balloon with your foot and it would feel as light as a feather. During this particular reserve game for Birmingham I knew I was struggling to run freely and didn't know exactly what was causing the problem. All I knew was that I needed to keep going in the hope that my body would loosen up and I could start to move with less restriction. But then someone passed me the ball and suddenly the problem I had with my running started to seem insignificant. I could see the ball at my feet and knew I was moving forward with it, but the shocking thing was that I couldn't really feel it. I was kicking the ball, but I couldn't really feel any contact. Or, to be more precise, I could feel it but it seemed as though I was kicking a balloon. That was the sensation I had, along with pins and needles in my feet, and as the game wore on things got no better. And just like kicking a balloon, every time I kicked the ball or passed it I couldn't be sure where it would end up.

It was scary, but what was even worse was the fact that I didn't feel I could say anything about it to anyone. The last thing I wanted was to be stopped from playing while I had more treatment, or was sent to hospital. I hoped that it was just a one-off feeling that would go away for ever, but I also knew that there seemed to be something else going on with my body. I had never felt like this in all the years I had been playing and training as a footballer. I was still a young man, but my body started to feel old. I didn't know why, but what I did know was that I had to carry on. I had to fight my way through whatever it was that was making everything feel so strange and make sure I came out the other side. Football had been my life, and despite all the aches, pains and pins and needles, I desperately wanted that life to continue.

CHAPTER TWELVE

HERO TO ZERO

Training had always been something I loved doing. Getting up and being paid to go out on a football pitch to run about for a couple of hours was a great way to spend a morning as far as I was concerned. I always appreciated the fact that I'd been born with certain talents that allowed me to go on and earn a very good living from playing a sport. I was always conscious of the fact that when I was on the training pitch on a Monday morning there was some poor guy out there slaving on a building site or working in a factory who would have paid me to be in my position. Perhaps it was because I had always been a naturally fit person that I enjoyed it so much. I wasn't too keen on things like runs or set-piece situations, but put a ball at my feet in a five-a-side or a practice match and I was in heaven. I would have run about all day as long as there was a football in front of me. But during that 1994/95 season with Birmingham the thought of getting up and driving the hour and twenty minutes to their training ground used to fill me with dread.

Although I wanted to put the bad experience of the reserve game behind me and hope that it would never happen again, I also realised that if I listened to my body I would hear it crying out to tell me there was something seriously wrong. Training used to make me feel good; I always felt fresh after I had finished. A couple of hours out of the day was nothing, and I often used to go on and do other things in the afternoon without feeling the least bit tired. But that started to change. Now, after driving back from Birmingham I would often get home and go straight to bed. Sometimes I actually slept right through to the next morning because I was so exhausted. I'd walk through the door, maybe have something to eat, and then head for the bedroom.

Within minutes of my head hitting the pillow I would be fast asleep. It didn't matter what was going on in the house, because no amount of noise from the kids or the television would wake me up.

I managed to get through those training sessions, but I know I must have looked bad sometimes, because I found it a struggle to move properly and co-ordinate my body in the way I needed to. I also felt shattered at the end of them, even if they hadn't been particularly demanding. I would sit in the dressing room totally drained by the effort I had put in, and with aches and pains making my body feel tight and uncomfortable. Most of the problems I got tended to focus on the right side of my body, just as they had done in previous years. The hamstrings, the calf and groin injuries – the vast majority were on the right. I thought nothing of it when they were happening, but because I had started to feel so strange in recent months I suppose I began to try to analyse things a bit more in my head. Perhaps I had a weakness somewhere in my back that was causing a problem? Back injuries are notorious for being difficult to sort out, and they can also have a knock-on effect when it comes to other parts of your body. For example, I'd known players who had real trouble with their hamstrings and it had all been down to the fact that they had injured a nerve in their back. I began to wonder if something like that had happened to me. It was a possibility, and at that time I was ready to hang on to any explanation I could come up with in the hope that I would eventually get back to feeling the way I had in the past.

The strange thing was that after years of feeling frustrated and upset at picking up hamstring and calf injuries, I was now more concerned with the way my whole body was feeling and reacting. I started to experience trouble doing simple things, like walking to my car after training. My body felt tight, and sometimes I would have a slight limp. It made me recall an incident at the airport after a European game Manchester United played against Torpedo Moscow in the autumn of 1992, for which I'd managed to get myself back in the side. We were checking in on our way back to Manchester, and Brian Kidd, who had come into the club as Alex Ferguson's assistant, was behind me in the queue. 'What's the matter with you?' he asked. 'You're limping. Is there something wrong with your hip?' I thought it was a strange question because I hadn't noticed anything wrong. I didn't think I was walking any differently than I normally did, but Brian said I was swinging my right foot out as if my hip joint was injured. Whatever was going on with my leg soon settled down and the limp must have disappeared because nothing more was said about it.

I'd not really thought about the incident since, but because of the problems I'd had, the memory came back into my mind. Surely I couldn't have been carrying an injury for over two years? After all, like any other player who gets transferred to another club, I had to undergo a medical when I joined Birmingham from United. I'm sure the medicals players have nowadays are a lot more thorough and exhaustive than they were back then, though. I have to admit that when I did make the move I can't remember being given too many tests, even though my career at Old Trafford had been blighted my small injuries. I think clubs were probably more concerned with things like broken legs and cartilage damage from the past. I suppose I was put through the standard medical. There were certainly no specialists on hand to check me over, and I passed without any problems.

It was difficult enough trying to mask the way I felt in those early months of 1995, and it soon got to the stage where other injuries were beginning to occur again just as they had in the past. Barry Fry had clearly had enough of me and wanted to put an end to the situation. He'd made up his mind that I was no use to him or the team, and although I didn't ever take to him as a manager or a person, I could understand his position. I'd played only about a dozen games during the time I'd been with the club, I was on decent money, and Birmingham were playing their football in the Second Division, although they were challenging for promotion by early spring. I was called in for a meeting with Karren Brady where she spelt out the options I had if I stayed at the club. Basically I was told that I would be training with the apprentices if I didn't move on, and I would also be doing their jobs with them as well. It wasn't the best thing to hear, but at least I knew exactly where I stood and the club was prepared to give me a payment to settle the contract I had with them. There was also the chance to move down to Wycombe and play under Martin O'Neill for a few months, and I knew that if I could prove my fitness there it might lead to a contract with the Wanderers, or perhaps another side that might be interested. As ridiculous as it may seem, I still thought I could play football and that one day I would be able to recapture the sort of form I'd had in the past.

I'm not really sure what Martin O'Neill thought of me during the time I was at Wycombe. He'd done a fantastic job as manager, taking the club into the Football League and putting them on the map. It was a well-run outfit, but the ground still had a non-league feel to it, even though at the time Wycombe were in the same division as Birmingham. The club was moving in the right direction, and the people down there were good to me, but when I look back at my time with them I can't help feeling embarrassed. I played about ten minutes in one game and then had to come off. That was the first and last time the Wycombe fans saw me play, and they must have wondered what all the fuss was about. Even by my own injury-prone standards, I knew I'd reached a new low. I saw the season out as an injured player and knew that if I wanted to continue my career I was fast running out of options. For the first time since I was a kid I faced the prospect of entering the summer months without a club. I'd gone from hero to zero in a very short space of time.

That summer of 1995 was a funny time for me. When you've been used to living your life as a footballer and suddenly you don't have a club, it feels very weird. There's a lack of structure about your life. When you're with a club your summer break stretches from the final game in May to reporting back for pre-season training in July. As a player I knew there was about a six-week gap between finishing a season and starting training again. We always tried to make the most of those weeks, and that was when we had to take our holidays. It would invariably be baking hot when we all reported back for training, and the first day of pre-season was something I looked forward to. It was a bit like going back to school after your summer holidays when you were a kid. Everyone was catching up with each other and finding out what had gone on while we'd all been away. It might only have been a matter of weeks, but it was like meeting up with long-lost friends. Then there were all the jokes and pranks that went on. Football club dressing-room humour is often dark and a bit sick, but if you ask any professional what he misses most when he has to pack in the game, top of his list will be actually playing and not far behind will be the daily banter with his team-mates. It's the sort of thing you take for granted and never think about until it's gone.

I had never been the sort of player who always had to be at the heart of things. I was happy to take a back seat because that's my personality. If I had been in a band, I suppose I would have been the drummer. But like anyone else who has played the game for a living, I became part of a team and a group of people. I'd got used to having lots of people around me most of the time. As a player you spend big chunks of time with your team-mates. Virtually every other week you find yourself sharing a room with another player on away trips, and quite often there will be days when you are away as a group. Such a lifestyle breeds a feeling of togetherness, but that summer, after failing to make any impression at all at Wycombe, I suddenly felt very alone and isolated. Of course I had Jenny and the kids, and there were my brothers and other family, but it was my football family that I was missing. For the first time since leaving school I found myself without one, and it was a very disorienting and uncomfortable experience.

At the end of any season there are players who are transfer-listed by their clubs, or unattached players who are free agents. I knew that most of them would be younger than me and they would also be fit and raring to go if a team came in and offered them an opportunity. I decided that I had to try to make sure I gave myself at least a fighting chance of being able to compete if a manager saw me on the list and decided to take a gamble, so without a club or a regimented pre-season training programme, I started to do some basic fitness work. Every morning I pulled on a tracksuit and went for a run near my home. The strange thing was that I didn't feel too bad. I was still getting tired after I'd finished, but the actual running didn't seem to be such a slog. I think it was probably due to the fact that I was doing it all at my own pace and wasn't being pushed or monitored in the way I would have been if I had been with a club. I remember going for a run one day and seeing Eric Cantona out on his bike. He shouted and waved at me as I slogged my way down the road, and he must have wondered what the hell I was doing.

Eric still lived near us and by this time had become a huge star with United. He was the player who really sparked things for them, and I wish I'd had the chance to play alongside him for a while. I'd watched some of the matches he'd played and he was magnificent in them. Although I hadn't spoken to him since I left Old Trafford I guessed that he was still very much the same as he'd been when he first arrived. He never struck me as the sort of person who would change, no matter how big a star he became with a United team that was now reckoned to be the best in the country. They'd followed up their success in winning the Premier League title in 1993 by going one better the following season: while I was struggling in a Birmingham side that got relegated, United retained the league title and also won the FA Cup, beating Chelsea 4–0. But I knew it was no good looking back at what might have been. I had to concentrate on what I was going to do in the future.

Like most footballers, I'd hardly thought about what would happen once I stopped playing, even though Jenny had often tried to get me to talk about the subject. I think it's a fault with a lot of players, although it might be slightly different these days. I know a lot of people will say that with the salaries many Premiership players are on now, all they have to think about when they retire is counting their money. But believe me, even the best-paid player in the world will feel the same as someone who has earned his living with a club way down in the league. The common link is that neither of them wants to stop playing. It's the thing they enjoy most. You become a professional footballer to play football. Sure the money is great, but there is nothing like actually playing in a team every week. That's why players hate being injured and out of the side. I'm sure there are a few who are happy to take the money and run, not worrying too much if they are in the first team or not, but they are in a minority. With what had happened to me during the final months of my time at Birmingham and then at Wycombe, I reckoned I probably had only one more throw of the dice when it came to getting my career going. I just didn't know how I was going to go about it.

Jenny was very supportive that summer. In her own mind I think she knew that I'd reached the end of the road as a player. She was no football expert, but she'd seen the way my game had deteriorated over the past few years and how I had struggled with injuries. She could also see a physical change in me. I would come home each day aching and then go off to bed. It wasn't normal behaviour for a professional footballer. I'd always rested at certain times, but being spark out for hours on end wasn't normal, and if I didn't want to face up to the fact, Jenny certainly did. We discussed whether it might be time for me to call it a day, but I just couldn't bring myself to admit that I wasn't up to it any more. I kept on thinking that I was still only 31 years old; lots of players went on until at least their mid-thirties, and quite often beyond that. I knew I'd had a terrible time with injuries, I knew my body felt as if it was giving up on me at times, but despite all of that I wanted to carry on. I was like an alcoholic wanting one more drink, only in my case I wanted just one more game in which to prove myself.

It came in the shape of a phone call from Andy King, the Mansfield Town manager. He'd heard that I was unattached and looking for a club and wondered if I fancied playing a pre-season game for them on 7 August against Notts County in the Nottinghamshire FA County Cup. Mansfield were in what was called Division Three at the time, but that didn't matter to me. Neither did the money. All I wanted was a footballing lifeline, and Mansfield were throwing me one. It was the chance I'd been hoping for, and although I knew I wasn't in peak condition as I drove to the match in my car, I also believed that I had enough ability and know-how to see me through. And who knows, it might lead to a season playing in Division Three. I was prepared to do that. At least I would be playing again instead of being a forgotten man.

I came on as a substitute for a player called Stewart Hadley, but very soon after stepping on to the pitch I knew it was all over. I struggled. I struggled to run, I struggled to control the ball, and I struggled to pass it. I had no energy, my balance was all over the place, and the pace that used to be such a big part of my game just wasn't there. It wasn't so much that I was a shadow of my former self, I'd virtually disappeared altogether.

CHAPTER THIRTEEN

A SLICE OF REALITY

For once, my mind was in agreement with my body: they both told me I had reached the end of the road. I came off at the end of that Mansfield match knowing I wasn't up to it. I couldn't perform in the way I'd hoped I would be able to, and this time there was no coming back. I was supposed to be with Mansfield for a week on a trial basis, but I knew it wasn't worth me carrying on and wasting Andy King's time. After all those years of being able to run and kick a ball well enough to be a top-flight professional footballer, I was faced with the harsh reality: my career was over.

I came away from the ground feeling numb and drained. I remember driving home and shaking my head at the thought of what had just happened. I wondered how I must have looked out there on the pitch, because if I'd looked as bad as I'd felt it must have been embarrassing. I could just imagine the spectators thinking, that can't be the same Danny Wallace who used to play for United and Southampton. Didn't he used to be quick? Wasn't he the one who scored that goal of the season on television? I wondered what had happened to him. What's he doing here? They were the sort of questions I would have been asking myself in the circumstances.

What was wrong with me? If you looked at my medical record, all you would have seen was a string of the same sort of 'little' injuries – hamstring, groin, calf, back. Not exactly career-threatening, yet along with all those injuries there had been a general and steady decline in my overall fitness. My form had been poor on occasions, but during the last couple of years the thing I had been most aware of was the way I just wasn't physically able to do the most basic things without worrying about them. For instance, there were times when I knew I couldn't just burst down the wing because I was aware the effort would leave me exhausted. I didn't move in the same way as I used to because I was frightened that a hamstring might go, or my back might begin to play me up. And in the very last months of my playing career I was aware of something a lot more sinister: my body was literally seizing up on me. I still felt that wear and tear had a lot to do with it. I was simply too ignorant, or too naive, to think it could be a symptom of anything more serious, although I think Jenny had her suspicions.

I always had a lot of energy, but while I was at Birmingham that had changed. Coming home and going to sleep after training was one thing, but it was the little things that I think Jen noticed. I would sit watching television and look drained, for example, even though I wasn't doing anything. I was reluctant to get involved in things and spent most of my time sitting around. I think part of the reason was because I was feeling sorry for myself, but it's still true to say that I didn't really have the energy to act in any other way. Without knowing it, slowly but surely, my body was changing.

Jenny was at the Mansfield game. I think she could see from my expression just how I felt.

'That's it, Jen,' I told her. 'It's over. I really struggled out there and I know I can't go on pretending it's all going to come right for me. I'm going to have to stop playing.'

After all that had happened I thought we needed a holiday, so we went off to Jamaica. It was good for both of us, and gave us the chance to do some thinking about how we were going to cope now that I had made the decision to stop playing. I had earned good money as a player, but not enough to keep us in the lap of luxury. We had a modest house in Worsley which still had a mortgage, and we'd had to sell our house in Southampton during the time I was at Birmingham. Although we rented out the property while I'd been in the north, the money we got barely covered the mortgage we still had on it. In the end we decided to sell the house and swallow the loss we'd made, because during the time we had the place its value had gone down. We had some savings, but not that much, and because I had no qualifications at all there were very few jobs I could go out and get which would earn us any decent money. We talked about the possibility of trying to start a business, but neither of us was sure what sort of business it should be. As much as I loved football, I didn't really fancy trying to stay in the game as a coach or manager. I had toyed with the idea of one day maybe getting involved at the youth level, because I appreciated how important that had been in my career and how much I had enjoyed the coaching I'd been given, but once again I needed to take my coaching badges for that to become a reality, and it was something I saw myself doing a few years down the line rather than straight away. Besides, it wasn't likely to bring in a great deal of money.

We came back from our holiday without anything decided. It was a strange period because I wasn't used to being around the house during the day and I found it difficult finding things to do with my time. I didn't let anyone know that I'd packed in playing; instead I just dropped out of the football scene. I also began to feel a bit better physically than I had for some time, but looking at the situation now I think it was because I was giving my body a rest. Until then I had been trying to play and train all the time, which meant I didn't get any real time for my body to recover. Once I had stopped playing completely I started to feel better and less tired, but that didn't really help our finances, and after talking things through again Jen and I decided on a new venture.

We came up with the idea of starting a sandwich business which we could run from our own home. The idea was to make the sandwiches and sell them to garages and shops in the area. We got two of our friends to help us and bought a freezer van to use for the deliveries. Jenny did a health and hygiene course to find out exactly how you should prepare the food and we got the relevant certificates from the local authority to allow us to start trading. Within a month or so of having the idea we were off and running, and we started to do pretty well. Jenny also began doing cooked breakfasts, baked potatoes and pasta in individual containers, which went down a storm with the guys on building sites. It was hard work, but after putting a lot of our own money into the project it was good to know that at least it seemed to have taken off. We used to have to get up really early in the morning to prepare all the food and then box and package it up ready to go on the van and be distributed to the various places who were regular customers.

I was feeling pretty good physically at the time, due mainly to the fact that I'd had about six months' complete rest from football and training. Once I'd made the decision to stop playing I hadn't done any training at all, and I didn't see anyone from the football world. I still kept in touch with Incy, just as I had done since I left United, but I didn't go to watch any matches and I honestly don't think people knew whether I was still playing or not. After all, I hadn't really played very much during the past few years when I was with United and then Birmingham, so I don't think many people missed me.

Of course, as busy as I was, I missed not being a footballer any more. It was the thing I had wanted to do from the moment I realised I had some ability with a ball at my feet. I had always thought that when the time came I would be able to look back on a career during which I had played regularly and done myself justice, but that wasn't the case. Almost from the time I went to United in 1989 my career had gone downhill; the worst part of it was thinking about the amount of time wasted because of injuries. I suppose I felt a bit cheated. I'd had a great start to my career, and perhaps that spoilt me a bit; certainly I'd expected it to get even better after the move to Old Trafford. How wrong I was. I also felt a bit embarrassed, of course. I don't think the United fans ever really got the chance to see me at my best. As for the Birmingham fans, they must have wondered why on earth the club bought me in the first place. My time there was a real nightmare, and it hadn't helped having a manager who I really didn't like and had no respect for. I've got happy memories of Southampton and of United, despite the way things turned out for me there, but I can't really say the same about Birmingham. The fans were fine and they always gave the team great support. They were good to me as well, even if they didn't see too much of me. But the fact that I felt so bad physically during the time I was at St Andrews, coupled with having Barry Fry as a manager and the way it all ended for me, means my memories of those eighteen or so months are sour ones. Still, as bad as it was for me at times at Birmingham, I would happily have swapped having to make and sell sandwiches for the chance to go back and play football again.

The reality was that it was never going to happen, and instead Jenny and I put everything we could into the business. We'd spent a lot of money setting things up, preferring to use our savings instead of arranging a bank loan, but after a few months I found I just couldn't keep up with things. I started to feel really tired, not just for an hour or two during the morning or afternoon, but all day long. I wasn't much help to Jenny, because while she would be up before dawn preparing everything and then out for most of the day selling sandwiches and cooked food, I would be at home sleeping. To add to her workload, one of the friends who had been helping us had to drop out.

Apart from the tiredness, I'd also begun to notice other physical problems. My body began to feel heavy, and my right side felt particularly bad. Quite often my back would feel as if it had a knot in it, and there were other, more alarming problems. At times I had a feeling of pins and needles in my right hand and right foot in much the same way as I'd experienced during that reserve game for Birmingham when the ball had started to feel like a balloon. Jenny also noticed that I sometimes limped, as if there was something wrong with my hip, because my right leg would kind of swing out sideways and I had trouble walking. I knew I had a problem, I just didn't know what it was. I'd been used to having injuries during the time I was playing, but this was something else. And it was literally getting worse by the day.

With me feeling so tired and lethargic and Jenny having to cope with the business virtually single-handed, we knew we couldn't carry on. We decided we would have to pack the business in. The two of us sat down one evening and talked the whole thing through. I didn't know what was wrong with me, and neither did Jenny, but we both knew I was ill and that I wasn't really capable of getting a job. Jenny decided that she would have to go out to work again, even though she wasn't sure what she could do. She put together a CV and sent it off to a lot of different businesses before getting a reply from a telesales company. She hadn't done anything like it before, but in typical fashion she threw herself into it, and it wasn't long before she landed another job working in the men's department at British Home Stores. I think at one stage she had about three jobs on the go at once. She became the breadwinner for the family; she never seemed to stop working. But the truth was, we needed the money. We were also using our savings as well to make sure all the bills were paid. It was a really difficult time for us, and not for the last time Jenny came to the rescue.

I can't recall who it was, but one day someone asked me if I had a pension. I hadn't really given it any thought. I knew that the pension scheme I paid into with the Professional Footballers' Association usually matured when you were 35 years old, and at the time I was 32, so I assumed I would have to wait another three years before getting any money. But Jenny had other ideas, and when we talked about it she said I ought to find out if there was any way I could get it early, because the simple fact was we needed the money. Jenny made a call to the PFA and spoke to the deputy chief executive Brendan Batson, explaining what had happened and asking whether it was possible to receive my pension early. She was told that it was possible, but only if it could be proved that my career had been prematurely ended because of illness or injury. I needed medical evidence, and that meant a series of tests and check-ups would have to be carried out. I was more than happy to undergo any test they wanted me to have. In fact, I began to hope that they could give me some sort of explanation for what had been happening to me, and maybe help me sort myself out.

CHAPTER FOURTEEN

BOOZE AT TEN

When you play football as a professional your life is filled with routines. You train every day, you play matches at weekends, you generally have things planned and mapped out for you. In the months following my enforced retirement from football in August 1995 my days had never felt so empty; in the months that followed my diagnosis at the Alexandra hospital in March 1997, they felt even emptier. Jenny had her jobs, the kids had their school, but all I had were the four walls that surrounded me every day. Of course, I could have made things better for myself. I could have got out, I could have found a hobby to get involved in, I could have found out more about multiple sclerosis, I could have got in touch with fellow sufferers, I could have maybe used the fact that I was a former player to head some sort of charity campaign. But I didn't. Not because I couldn't, but because I chose not to. Instead, I preferred to wallow in my own little world. I refused to talk to people and didn't even want to see my mates, who had been such a regular part of my life during my playing days. They were people I had known for years, people I had grown up with, but the visits became less frequent, not because they didn't want to see me but because I couldn't be bothered to see them.

I retreated into myself and found it difficult to talk about what was happening to me, even to Jen. She tried to discuss it, but I put up barriers and refused to open up. She knew she would have to help me every day for the rest of my life, and I knew it too, but there was something in me that refused to accept the situation. I wasn't prepared to own up even to having the illness, and I hardly told anyone about it. My brothers were told, though, and my parents. My mum took it badly and was in tears when she heard. Like most people, she didn't fully understand the disease and the forms it can take. Saying someone has MS can be as shattering and frightening as saying they have cancer, but in both cases it doesn't have to mean a death sentence. I think the thought of seeing her son go from being someone who had boundless energy on the football pitch and was always full of life to being a physical shadow of himself was naturally upsetting for her. But I know that her and Jenny became very close at the time and mum was a big help to her. It's something Jen has always appreciated and they are still very close to this day. I told Paul Ince as well, but nobody else from the world of football. Our friends found out through Jenny, but I never wanted to talk about it to anyone. If people found out, that was fine, but I wasn't going to tell anyone. The children knew too. They didn't really understand, although they could see how badly I'd deteriorated, and the process had happened quite literally in front of their eyes. Little Thaila was already at a nursery school because it was thought he had a speech difficulty; sending him to nursery early was recommended to help bring him up to speed. That was probably a blessing for Jenny because it meant she knew he would be at school all day and out of the house. She was working shifts, which suited her because it made things a little more flexible. Remi and Elisha were also out of the house all day at school, which meant I was at home and alone, with plenty of time to think and sink deeper into a depression.

The strange thing about being depressed is that you don't really know about it. Everything seems pretty normal to you and there are no obvious signs, although I'm sure there are to others. With Jenny and the children out of the house I found myself sitting around every day looking at the four walls of our lounge and going over and over what had happened. There was no feeling of relief any more; it had been replaced by desperation. I never once during this period tried to face the problem head on and think positively about the future. I left that sort of thing to Jenny. If I'd treated her badly in the past by going off for nights out with my mates and cheating on her with other girls, it was nothing compared to what I must have put her through for quite a time after finding out about the MS. Jenny is a strong lady with more resilience than I will ever have, but how she didn't become ill because of me I will never know. Not only was she working virtually around the clock with different jobs to earn money for the family, she was looking after the children and a husband who hardly spoke to her. When I did talk it was often to shout or show off. It was as if I thought that after being diagnosed I had the right to act and behave as badly as I wanted to the woman who loved and cared for me. Jenny was very good about it and took all the stick and my bad moods, but I'm sure there must have been times when she had to bite her tongue. She did have a go back sometimes, and who could blame her? I remember her lashing out at me on a couple of occasions through sheer frustration. She had come home after looking after people with disabilities that were far worse than mine and then had to put up with me. But considering the way I was behaving she managed to keep things together really well. I'm sure she must have wanted to tell me exactly where to go at times and not be so self-pitying. After all, she had to deal with some very bad cases of disability at work and knew that all of those people were trying as hard as they could to make a life for themselves despite their physical problems. Then she had to come home to me and all my brooding.

Certain things began to become a problem for me. I found that I could no longer lift anything that was a bit heavy, and I also lost my balance on occasions. I would also bump into things for no apparent reason. I could walk across a room, and if there was a table or chair in my path it was odds-on that I would clip it as I went past. It didn't seem to matter that I had a clear view of it and was aware it was there, I would still hit the thing. Still, instead of trying to cope and making plans for the future, all I wanted to do was stick my head in the sand. It was crazy behaviour, and when I think about it now I realise how stupid I was, but I was struggling to cope with the way I was feeling.

Despite the pins and needles in my right hand and sometimes in my leg, I was still able to move around, it was just that my movement had become slower. Sometimes I limped as well. I was very conscious of it, and that was why I didn't like to leave the house. People still made the trip up from London to see us, and although I wasn't as social as I had been in the past, Jenny and my friends told me it would do me good to get out and act normally. When we were younger we all used to love going to clubs, and one weekend it was decided we'd go into Manchester for something to eat and then go on to a club. When we got to the nightclub there was a huge line of people behind a roped-off area waiting to go in, and as I turned to join the queue I suddenly lost my balance and toppled over. My leg had kicked out and I couldn't do anything about it. I found myself on the pavement looking up at all the punters and hearing them muttering about me being drunk. But I hadn't even had a drink. It was simply the MS: my body had knotted up and I was kicking around on the ground unable to get myself up. Jenny and my mates tried to help me, but I started shouting at them to leave me alone. I was angry, embarrassed and frustrated. In the end I had to agree to let them haul me to my feet or I would have been spinning around on that pavement all night like an out-of-control break-dancer because I physically didn't have the capability to do anything about it. It was hopeless, and I felt so helpless. My mates were the very people I should have opened up to at that time, but it didn't happen. Instead, I found a new friend, and it came in a bottle.

I had always liked a drink, even when I was playing, and although I sometimes had a bit too much, it never got out of control. My football meant too much to me; I would never have put it in jeopardy by boozing to excess on a regular basis. I had gone out with my mates after matches and had a good drink, but I was young and fit, and I never missed a day's training because of drinking. I know some players have gone off the rails even though they've had great careers, but that was never going to be me. I was a social drinker; when I was training during the week or there was a game coming up, I never went near the stuff. I valued what I did too much and I always wanted to be as fit as I could be when I went on the pitch. I think drinking was much more part of the football culture when I first went into the game, and as I've already said, it was the done thing to stay behind after a match and have a few beers with your friends, family and the rest of the team after a match. It was Jenny's favourite part of match day. There was always a really nice atmosphere at Southampton and United after matches. When I was at Old Trafford the kids would also come because the club had a crèche for the young ones while their mums watched the match. It was a welcome idea, and it made Saturdays a nice day out for everyone.

After games I often liked to carry on drinking with my mates and go out to a club or two while Jenny went home. Most times she didn't really mind, though there were occasions when she got fed up with my antics. After we moved to Manchester she put her foot down several times, and once, when she had arranged to see some friends of her own, Jenny ordered our baby-sitter to make sure I didn't leave the house and sneak out for a night on the town. I also remember waking up early one morning and realising that I was lying on the floor of my lounge stark naked. I'd been out the night before and must have returned home the worse for wear. Apparently Jenny was so upset with the state of me that she stripped me and left me downstairs to teach me a lesson. I woke up shivering. When I realised where I was I suddenly became aware that I had no clothes on. I got up and knew it was daylight because the curtains were open, and not only could I see out but the postman, who was delivering letters, could see in. He must have wondered what the hell I was doing.

Despite instances like that, though, I was not a boozer. Certainly the idea of sitting at home drinking on my own would never have entered my head. But things changed when I had to pack the game in and cope with MS, and as I said, I made a new friend by the name of Brandy. I can't say exactly when it was, but for some reason as I sat watching the television one morning I decided I wanted a drink. The strange part was that I didn't think it was an odd thing to be doing, even though it was still morning and I'd just come back from a school run. I remember shuffling over to the cabinet on the other side of the room, pulling out a bottle of cognac and pouring myself a large glass of the stuff. I sat down and drank it before getting up and pouring myself another. Suddenly I felt better than I had done for weeks. It was as if something nice had happened to me for once after all the shit I felt had been thrown at me. It also made me feel physically more relaxed, and as the alcohol wandered through my veins, the aches and pains that had become constant companions decided to have a rest. It felt good. So good, in fact, that I poured myself a third drink. By this time I was lying back on the couch having decided that life wasn't so bad after all.

The booze helped me to feel better about myself and see things more clearly – or so I thought. In reality it did nothing of the sort, but my new friend was very persuasive and had soon convinced me that as long as we were together my world would be a better place. After having a few drinks I fell asleep and woke up just in time to realise that I had to pick Thaila up from school. The aches and pains were back again as I washed up my glass, and as an added bonus I also had a throbbing head. That night I had another drink as Jenny arrived home from work before getting ready to go out to a second job. I don't know if she noticed that I was nicer to her than I had been in a while, but if she did I'm sure she wouldn't have been happy that the change in my usual mood had been brought about by my new friend.

I soon got used to having my new mate with me from about ten in the morning. It quickly became a routine, and one that was very easy to slip into. Jenny was working different shifts with the NHS, but quite often she would be out from early in the morning until late afternoon or evening. I used to take young Thaila to school in the morning and then come home to my four walls and my thoughts. Those thoughts grew darker as the days and weeks went on, and the drinking got heavier. Moreover, the feeling I got from it wasn't always as good as it had been that very first time. Sometimes, instead of giving me a lift it had the reverse effect and I started to feel unhappy, but most of the time it seemed to help. Sometimes I would sit for two or three hours just sipping gently at the brandy in my hand. I became used to the drink, and because of that I was able to stay sober for longer before the full effects started to kick in.

Lots of those days I spent at home alone were the same. I had my little routine and I kept to it. I would drink and think until I got too tired and had to sleep for an hour or two. As I drank I would go over all sorts of things in my head and sometimes have conversations with myself, all of them along similar lines. I found it easy to talk when nobody was around me, yet when it came to talking to Jenny and opening up in the same sort of way, I just wasn't able to do it. Usually by the time she got home I'd sobered up and wasn't in the same sort of mood I had been during the day, when I talked to myself about the MS that had taken over my body, about having my career taken away from me because of it; I talked to myself about the way I just loved kicking a ball around as a kid and the fact that I was so sure I was going to make it, and about the good times when I was flying with Southampton and it looked as though my career would go on for ever. I smiled at the thought of the day when I made my debut for Southampton, and the clip around the ear I got from Lawrie for not calling him boss. Sometimes I would drink and watch a video on the television. I had tapes of some of the games I had played in and enjoyed watching familiar faces flit across the screen. I would smile when I saw someone like Jimmy Case crunching into a tackle and then making a goal for me. It made me remember the time at Newcastle in the mid-eighties when I was sent off for the first time in my career, thanks to mistaken identity. Jimmy had gone hurtling into a tackle with Newcastle's John Anderson and went through the poor guy like a missile. Players from both sides went flying in, pushing and shoving, but by this time Jimbo had fled the scene and was as far away from all the action as he could be. The referee came over and booked me even though I hadn't made the tackle and I was a different colour to Jimmy. Later on I got a second yellow for a different offence, which meant I was sent off. The club appealed on my behalf and Jimmy went along with me to the FA. I think they were a bit embarrassed by the whole thing. The only reason I could think of for the referee's action was that we both had moustaches at the time.

Little things like that used to give me a lift, but they were invariably followed by darker moods during which I started to blame the world for the problems I had. The thing I resented most was the fact that I felt my career had been snatched away from me and it hadn't been a sudden thing. It had happened over a period of years, and because of that it had felt like a lingering death. People just thought I had become a poor player and that I was a waste of money. I knew that both Remi and Elisha had had to put up with a few remarks from other kids at their school because of what had happened at United. Elisha actually had someone come up to her and say that I was a rubbish footballer, and she got into a fight with the boy who had said it. Remi was at the same school and getting similar stick because of my form with United, and some of the comments got a bit racist. Like his little sister, Remi stood up for me and got into fights because of it, even though at the time I wasn't exactly being the best dad in the world to either of them.

That was another part of the drinking: it made me take stock of all sorts of things in my life. I realised I hadn't ever really been there for either Remi or Elisha. I wished I had been more involved with Remi and talked more to him, but I didn't, mainly because I was always too self-centred. I was only concerned with playing football, and then when I did have time off I tended to spend it with my mates, not with my kids. I know now that I was wrong, but you can never turn the clock back and change things.

At about the time I started drinking, Remi, who was only fourteen, decided to start sampling another sort of drug to the one his dad was pumping down his throat. Unsurprisingly, with all the upheaval there had been at home, he'd found himself getting less attention. Remi had always loved his mum – they were just as much friends as they were parent and child – but Jenny wasn't around the house as much as she had been because she was out at work, and my relationship with Remi had never been that close. He started to hang around with a group of friends and not only made himself ill after drinking a strong beer, he also sampled cannabis. The situation soon got out of control and came to a head when he was expelled by his school for trying to sell the stuff to other kids. It was a situation that called for me to be in control and act as a dad should do. I should have been able to talk to him and find out why he'd done what he did, but it never happened. I think he was hanging out with people he thought he could communicate with, and who would listen to him. It was something he got precious little of from me because I was so wrapped up in my own world.

The drinking certainly began to fill a gap in my life, and I started to hit the bottle more heavily. Jenny was not stupid, and although I probably thought I was hiding things from her, the truth was that she knew what I was up to. For a start, I think the number of empty bottles was a pretty good giveaway, and I know she came home on more than one occasion and could smell the booze on my breath. Jenny got into the habit of ringing me while she was at work and asking me to do things around the house. It was her way of keeping a check on me while she was out, knowing that if I had to do little jobs I wouldn't be sitting on a couch with a glass of brandy in my hand. Sometimes it would be to ask me to phone someone, or to put some washing in the washing machine; other times she might ask me to do some cooking and would leave the recipe for a particular meal in the kitchen before she went to work. But I still managed to get the brandy down my neck, and by this time I wasn't really bothered if Jenny knew about it or not, because I wasn't going to stop. The fact was, I liked drinking. It gave me something to do, and most times it helped me to feel better about myself.

It seemed as though I was getting worse physically, and because of that I think I began to hit the bottle even more. It wasn't a good situation, and in my sober moments I realised that, but I didn't have the will or the self-discipline to stop. One day, after taking Thaila to school I got back to the house and immediately poured myself a drink. I'm not even sure if I'd had anything to eat that morning, but it didn't seem to matter. Once I had a drink in my hand I felt better. I took up my usual position on the sofa, and apart from going to the toilet I pretty much stayed there for the next six hours sipping brandy, until it was time to pick Thaila up. I got in the car, drove to his school, and then drove back home without ever thinking that I must be way over the limit. I could easily have killed both of us. I'm sure I wasn't driving properly, but I managed to make it home unscathed, and I'm sure I did the same sort of thing on other occasions as well. I wasn't drinking bottles of brandy at a time, and I never got to the stage where Jenny came home and found me paralytic because of the booze, but I did drink steadily and on a daily basis.

It wasn't an easy thing for her to have to cope with on top of everything else, and she provided a safety net when it came to Thaila being picked up, because quite often she would do it herself, or she would get our baby sitter Alex to collect him as well, knowing that I might well have been drinking during the day.

I had developed a serious problem, but I didn't want to admit it.

CHAPTER FIFTEEN

TUNNEL VISION

The booze became a permanent fixture in my life because it helped me cope with the situation I found myself in. It made me feel better mentally and eased the physical pain. The drink also helped me to stay in the tunnel I had created for myself. I'd already done a pretty good job of staying in that tunnel and cutting off the rest of the world, but what I was also doing at the same time was cutting off my family.

When Remi was expelled for dealing drugs at his school I was angry and upset with him. I couldn't believe that he would get involved in something like that, and neither could his mother. We were both devastated by the news, but my way of dealing with it was to shout and scream at him. Of course he'd done something wrong and it was stupid, but at the same time he was just a fourteen-year-old kid. He'd made a mistake, and at the time my only reaction to what had happened was anger. I didn't try to sit him down and talk to him. I didn't ask why he'd done it, what he was thinking. I wasn't really there for him as a father in the way I should have been because I was more interested in wallowing in my own problems instead of helping my son with his.

If I'm honest, I have to admit that I had never been that close to Remi. I had never given him the sort of time and attention I should have. When he was younger I was more interested in doing what I wanted to do than in sitting down with him and talking. I know a lot of people automatically seemed to think that because he was my son he would be good at football, but he never was that good. He was better at rugby. That didn't bother me, but I'd never told him that. Little things like that can affect a young boy as he's growing up. I didn't realise it at the time, but he's since told me about the pressure he felt to follow in my footsteps. I should have known things like that. I should have been a friend as well as a father, but it never happened simply because I couldn't be bothered. I didn't take the time to do the right things for him, and then, just when he needed me most as a young teenager, I went missing again. Not physically, but mentally.

It wasn't that I didn't care about Remi, it was that I didn't care enough. It was Jenny who went to a two-hour meeting at his school to hear all about what had gone on and why Remi was going to be asked to leave, and it was Jenny who had to sort out getting him into another school. She had always been closer to him than I had, and at least she gave him her time and attention. The trouble was, Jen was out of the house a lot of the time earning money for all of us. Considering that Remi was at home with me and my terrible moods, it was no wonder that he decided he'd be better off on the streets with his mates. At least he got some conversation out of them, which was more than he ever got with me.

Most times my way of communicating with Remi was to shout at him and have rows. It wasn't just the booze that made me so bad-tempered, it was also the general resentment towards the world that I felt at the time. Poor Remi just seemed to bear the brunt of it on so many occasions, although I also had a go at Elisha and Jenny as well. If I'd done what I was asked to do by Jen and cooked a meal that she'd given me the recipe for, I used to go berserk if the kids tried to get out of doing the washing-up. It was almost as if I was trying to pick fights with all three of them for the least thing. They must have dreaded meal times in our house because none of them knew what might send me off on a rant. I think they all tried to avoid me as much as they could in the hope that it would prevent a scene. Jenny has since told me that they all felt as though they were treading on eggshells with me back then. I never got really violent, but I was abusive, and spurred on by the daily drinking I began to care less and less about what they thought. The only thing I really cared about was me and what had happened to me.

I still thought I was being discreet with my drinking, but Jenny was well aware of it, and I think the kids had cottoned on as well. As far as Jen was concerned it was something that she hoped I would come out of. She could understand how upset and depressed I was at what had happened, and she knew that having my career wrenched away from me had been a devastating experience. I think at first she thought a drink or two might get me through a few bad weeks, but the weeks soon turned into months and Jenny knew that I was having more than just one or two glasses while she was at work. She did confront me on several occasions and told me that I should stop, but although there was some screaming and frustration I think that somehow she hoped that I would stop before it became too late. It must have been a terrible time for her.

Jenny is a strong and determined woman, but coming home to see her husband glassy-eyed because of drink must have put a strain on her. The safety valve she had was being so heavily involved in working for the NHS. She loved the job and got tremendous satisfaction out of helping the disabled people she cared for. I think work took on a whole new meaning for her once she knew I had MS, and her experience and training certainly helped her cope with me. The difference was that the people she dealt with in her working life were all grateful and willing to put themselves out. When she got home to her husband I was quite often sullen, bad-tempered and unwilling to put myself out in any way at all. I didn't want any light in the dark tunnel I had built for myself. I was happy to shut it all out and mope around the house.

When I was there on my own at home during the day, the only real contact I had with the outside world was when I took Thaila to school in the morning and then picked him up in the afternoon. Our friends had continued to call to try to get me to go for nights out with them, but I always found an excuse, and in the end I think they realised it was a pretty hopeless task. I had gone from being very sociable and having lots of friends around the house on a fairly regular basis to not wanting to see anyone. The more the days went on with me not seeing anyone, the more I got used to the sort of life I had made for myself. I had become a virtual recluse, and I liked it that way. I didn't want to be seen out and about because I was so aware of the way I must look. I didn't want anyone recognising me and asking me questions. It wasn't as if I couldn't have gone out for a walk, because I was still capable of doing that. But I tended to limp slightly, and walking was becoming more of an effort.

The other thing that concerned me was the fact that in many ways I was still learning to live with MS, and it still had some surprises for me. I had good days and bad days. The good days were when I was more in control of things and could cope better with the way my body felt; the bad days were when I suddenly didn't seem to have any control at all and I would be in pain or perhaps lose my balance. Just to add to my discomfort, I didn't really take anything to control my condition. There were drugs on the market, and I was told that some of them would help to ease the condition for me, but I'd always hated taking pills and tablets. I did take one particular drug for a while but had to stop when I found they affected my vision and made me feel sick.

Instead, I preferred to hit the bottle because I felt comfortable with it. I also thought I was in control and that my drinking had not got out of hand. If I'd taken a step back I would have been able to see how ridiculous that was. Drinking brandy on your own at ten in the morning is not normal behaviour, neither is trying to conceal the fact that you have been on the booze. Jenny has told me what a worrying time it was for her, and she must have been under tremendous strain. She had a very responsible job, plus a couple of other part-time ones on the go as well, a husband who might well have been drinking himself to death for all she knew, and on top of all that three kids to look after, one of whom had already had a brush with drugs. I'm more convinced now than ever that a lesser person would have cracked up under the pressure or just run away from it all. There was I, sinking into depression and feeling sorry for myself, while at the same time she was working herself silly to keep the family together and care for someone with MS who didn't seem to appreciate anything that was being done for him.

To say I was selfish is being kind. I acted and behaved like a complete bastard to my wife and to my kids. Instead of trying to pull myself together and appreciate not only what I had at the time but also what a great life I'd had until the illness came along, I chose to blame and resent everyone and everything. It was me kicking out against the world, and it couldn't have been a pretty sight. I wasn't the only person in the world with multiple sclerosis, and there were other sufferers in far worse a condition. Some of them had a death sentence hanging over their heads. I may have had the illness, but if I approached it in the right way I would be able to cope and build a different sort of life. The trouble was, I instinctively didn't want to accept that my old life was over. I wanted to cling on to what it was like, not to accept the position I was in. When pain came, instead of taking properly prescribed medication, I took my own in the form of brandy.

Although I'd managed to keep most people at arm's length and my house wasn't as busy as it had been in the past, I was happy to see my elder brother Clive when he decided to travel up to see us during this dark period in my life. He managed to raise my spirits a bit as we talked over some of the days when we were both kids, and about some of the people we had known. Jenny was probably relieved to have him around as well because the atmosphere in the house was better and it helped ease some of the pressure off her shoulders. All three of us had a few drinks, and we also had some laughs – something that had been missing from the house for a while. I felt pretty relaxed and was enjoying everything, but then I started talking about the MS, and for the first time since I'd been diagnosed the mask I'd been holding up in front of me slipped. Suddenly I felt my eyes welling up with tears and I began to cry.

'Why me, Clive?' I managed through the sobbing. 'Why me? What did I do to deserve it? Why did it have to happen?'

I think it was the booze that made me so emotional, but at the same time I knew I was letting my true feelings come out. I did want to know why it was me who had contracted the illness. I did want to know what I'd done to deserve getting it, and having my football career prematurely ended because of it. I knew I wasn't the only person with MS, but that was no consolation. I had never felt so low in all my life, and despite the love and care people like Jenny wanted to give me, I had never felt so alone either. I knew I had physical problems, but I was also sinking lower and lower mentally as I struggled to come to terms with my life. The drinking had now become second nature to me, a way of life. After all those years of football, the booze had helped fill the void, and I'd made a close friend of it. But something inside told me the friend was now my enemy. I knew that if I didn't do something about it I would end up in a much worse state.

That night with Clive and Jen I took the first small step towards emerging from the gloom of my tunnel, but I still wasn't sure what the light at the end would bring.

CHAPTER SIXTEEN

MANAGING TO GET A LIFE

I'm not exactly sure how long I was drinking heavily, but I think it lasted for about eighteen months, and stopping was a gradual process. I didn't just wake up one morning and decide that I'd had my last drink. In fact, I've never actually stopped drinking alcohol. I still have a drink or two today, but I'm sensible about it, just like most people are. There's nothing abnormal about my consumption these days. It used to be a case of me guzzling the stuff down during the day as I sat in an empty house, but after the dark period I'd spent in that tunnel I found that I wanted some light. The daytime drinking stopped, and although I still had a glass in the evening with Jenny, I didn't have the reliance on it I'd had before. I don't think it's too dramatic or overstating the case to say that I might well have ended up dead had I carried on the way I was going. I've heard and read things about alcoholism, and although I don't think I had the full-blown thing, I'm convinced I went close to it. If I hadn't eased off in the way I did there would only have been one outcome: I would have gone steadily downhill. Not drinking during the day helped me to think more clearly. But don't get me wrong, I hadn't changed completely overnight. I was still a miserable, self-pitying, self-centred ex-footballer who thought the world was against him, but at least I was having those thoughts while I was sober and not drunk.

Despite drinking heavily for a long period of time I'd still managed to function pretty normally, or at least as normally as the MS would allow me to. By that I mean that I was able to do things like helping to cook a meal, or maybe tidy up bits and pieces around the house. I didn't do too much while I was at home, and that was probably one of the main reasons why I slipped into the brandy habit. It filled a gap and made the day go quicker. Jenny's phone calls and her little lists of things that had to be done occupied me to some extent, but quite often I wouldn't do what she'd asked me to simply because I couldn't be bothered. It was probably also a way of me saying that I would only do what I wanted to do, and nobody else was going to tell me how to live my life. If I wanted to sit around all day and look at the four walls of our lounge, then I would do just that.

The one thing that I was conscientious about was taking Thaila to school and picking him up every day. I bitterly regret the fact that some of those trips home must have been made while I was over the limit after drinking too much brandy during the day, and I just thank God that I was lucky enough not to have an accident. The thought that I could possibly have killed my own son because of my boozy ways sends a shudder down my spine whenever I think about it. But even during those miserable days I always enjoyed having Thaila around. He actually managed to make me laugh with some of his antics when he was in the house, and it was good for me to have time with him. It was the sort of time I had never given to Remi or his sister Elisha when they were both a similar age.

Getting to know Thaila and doing things like reading to him seemed to be just about the only good thing that had happened since my diagnosis. He seemed to be a happy, outgoing little boy. We'd been warned by the school about a problem with his speech, but that turned out to be a false alarm, and there was no doubt that mixing with other kids and having the structure of being at school every day helped him come on. The thing I noticed most about him as he played around the house in the afternoons was that, in marked contrast to the way I felt every day, he had a genuine love of life and was enthusiastic about everything. Thaila always seemed to be bubbly and eager to please; I was pretty much always miserable and couldn't wait to jump down the throats of Jenny, Remi and Elisha. Most of the time it was about nothing at all, and when it came to Remi I constantly seemed to be on at him over silly little things.

After he had been expelled for dealing drugs Jenny had managed to get him into another school, but he hated being there and couldn't wait to leave. He was no different to me in that respect, because I never wanted to be at school. You could hardly say that I was academic when I was at West Greenwich. But at least I had a driving ambition to be something; I wasn't sure that Remi had any idea what he was going to do once he did leave. I should have sat him down and asked him, paid more attention to what was happening in his life, but I didn't. Years earlier it had been my football and going out with my mates which had been more important to me; then, when I got a second stab at actually being the father Remi deserved, I cocked it up again because I was too busy wallowing in a mixture of self-pity and booze. One day on the way home from school with Thaila I saw Remi hanging around on a street corner with some of his mates. It was the middle of the afternoon and it was clear he had been bunking off school. I went absolutely mad and told him he wasn't going to be allowed to leave the house and see his mates, but once again I didn't bother to talk to him in a sensible way, which might just have made him understand how important it was for him to get a decent education and not spend his time hanging around street corners.

I don't know whether I was harbouring any guilt about not being able to relate to Remi, or about the way I'd neglected him as a dad, but I found myself wanting to make sure I didn't make the same mistake twice. I started to spend a lot of time with Thaila, and for the first time I actually took a proper interest in one of my children. Don't get me wrong, I loved all of my children, but I'd been the absent father to the older two because I'd been so wrapped up in my football, leaving Jenny to get on with things. I think they both enjoyed the fact that I was a footballer when they were young, but it brought problems for both of them. I've mentioned the playground fights when my career started to go downhill at United, but there were other things as well. I didn't know it at the time, but Remi has since told me that he felt very unsure of people when he was a kid, because he believed so many of them only wanted to know him because of who his dad was. It couldn't have been very nice to find out that one of the boys at school only wanted to be your friend because he was interested in finding out more about your dad and what went on at United. He even had a teacher who wasn't particularly nice to him in the classroom, but then had the cheek to ask if Remi could get her a ticket for a game at Old Trafford. It's something Jenny guarded against too. Soon after we moved to Manchester she became friendly with a girl who asked Jen what I did for a living. She told her I was a bricklayer because she didn't want to get involved with talking about United and football, and she thought it made sense not to let on who I was and what I did. If she met someone new it was better that they became friends because they liked and got on with each other, rather than have someone clinging to Jen because they wanted to know someone whose husband happened to be a footballer. Elisha had to cope with people knowing who I was as well, but I think she was quite proud to have a dad who played for United. She once hung around me after a game as all the fans swarmed around me and the rest of the players asking for autographs. 'Come on, Dad, come on, Dad,' she kept saying, and I thought she was desperate for us to get away and go home, but apparently what she really wanted to do was let everyone within earshot know that she was my daughter and I was her dad.

The time I spent with Thaila definitely had a therapeutic effect on me. I had to be more responsible instead of just thinking about myself. It was what I needed at the time. Having to look after Thaila not only took my mind off the MS, I think it also slowly began to turn me into a better person. As I started to leave the booze behind me he was beginning to get quite big. He was only about four or five, but he was full of life and I had to try and keep up with him. I knew I couldn't do the thing I would most like to do – kick around a ball with him – but I was able to read and have little conversations with him. I did have a ball in the garden that he played with and I sometimes put my foot to it, but I couldn't take a proper kick because I knew I would have ended up flat on my face. It was another indication to me of just how far away my days as a player actually were.

It was by this stage getting on for a decade since I had made that trip up from Southampton to Manchester with Bob Higgins to meet

Alex Ferguson and Martin Edwards, though it seemed a lot longer than that. While my career went downhill, Fergie and United just seemed to go from strength to strength. By the summer of 1999 they'd won five Premier League titles, four FA Cups, a League Cup and the Champions League. I would have loved to be involved in all that success. To be honest, just getting to another cup final would have been brilliant. But I had to come to terms with the fact that I had stopped being a top footballer a long time ago. Way back in those United days in fact. At least I now knew that all the injuries and problems had been real. I hadn't faked them or taken the easy way out, as I'm sure some people thought at the time. They were legitimate injuries, and I was now more convinced than ever that a lot of them had a connection with my MS. The illness might not have been full-blown at that time, but I knew how my body felt towards the end of my time at Old Trafford, and the sensation of having my legs feel so tired and heavy in some reserve games wasn't just because of a lack of match fitness. I'd tried so hard to make things work out, and in some of the drunken conversations I had with myself I did wonder aloud whether the effort I put in and the strain I felt at the time had anything to do with speeding up the onset of the disease. I know I can never prove it, but I can look back and remember how I felt both physically and mentally.

Professionally speaking, joining United was the biggest thing to happen to me, and although it didn't work out the way they or I would have liked, I still love the place. United aren't just a club, they're an institution. People from all over the world have heard about them. When they stepped out on to the pitch in Barcelona to take on Bayern Munich on that May evening in 1999 I was sitting on my sofa at home reliving some of my Old Trafford memories. The good ones, like the day I signed and was introduced to the home crowd before that match with Millwall, and the fantastic night when we won the FA Cup final replay against Crystal Palace. And the bad ones: the feeling that even after only a year at the club my career was slipping away from me; the injuries that became part of my everyday life; the knowledge that there were at least two or three players ahead of me when it came to claiming a first-team place. The writing was on the wall for me, but it was as if I ended up bashing my head against that wall in an effort to become a regular first-team player at the club. The harder I tried, the worse it got. I always felt I'd let myself down and underperformed during my time with the club, and when I left I felt embarrassed. I almost wanted to slink away and not be noticed. I'd gone there with high hopes of joining some of the legends I'd looked up to as a kid, and because I had done so well with Southampton in the First Division I had every reason to believe I could go to Old Trafford and make a name for myself. But after that first season and the win against Palace, things just went rapidly downhill for me.

I would be lying if I said I wasn't jealous of the United players when they walked out to face Bayern Munich, especially as that year the Champions League final could not have been more exciting or dramatic. When Teddy Sheringham got the equaliser with a couple of minutes to go I wanted to jump out of my seat and celebrate with him. Of course there was no way I could manage to do it, and anyway, I hardly had time to get over the fact that United had got themselves back in it at the death before Ole Gunnar Solskjaer grabbed the winner in the last seconds of the match. It was incredible, an amazing achievement for the club and Alex Ferguson. When I thought back to all the pressure he had been under when I joined them, the night seemed even more remarkable. His reaction after the match, when the television cameras caught him grinning and looking relieved, reminded me of that final against Palace in 1990. Winning that match had killed off all the talk about when he was going to lift his first trophy, or whether he was capable of producing a winning Manchester United team. Beating Bayern was the same in many ways. He must have gone to United from Aberdeen knowing that Matt Busby was a legend and had won it all as a manager at Old Trafford, including the biggest club prize of them all, when his side beat Benfica to take the European Cup in 1968. No United manager had managed to do that since, but Fergie had slowly built a squad good enough to do it.

The only real link I had with it was Ryan Giggs, the only one of that new crop of United talent to have claimed a regular place in the side before I departed for St Andrews and those bad days at Birmingham. I was really pleased for him, not only because he was a friendly guy, but also because he worked hard at his game. He had been blessed with phenomenal talent, but he knew that wasn't enough if he was going to go on and be a great player. Ryan knew all about the work ethic, and with someone like Fergie in charge it was unlikely any of his players would forget it. He always used to instil into his teams the need to work and be competitive from the first whistle to the last. If that happened and you had good players, then the likelihood was that you would come out on top. Fergie was also a master tactician; he knew how to set his teams up. People knew exactly what their jobs were and what was expected of them. He must have been absolutely delighted to have pulled it off and beaten Bayern Munich. All managers love winning, and in 1999 Fergie won the biggest one of all.

So of course I was happy for them, for Fergie and for the club, but I was sad for myself. I'm not saying I would have been one of those players had I steered clear of injuries and not been hit by multiple sclerosis, because by May 1999 I was 35 years old. My best days would surely have been behind me. But, how I would have loved the chance to sample a match of that importance and be fully involved in it! If things had taken off for me at Old Trafford it is quite likely that I would have been in the thick of it when they were winning league titles and cups, just as people like Steve Bruce, Incy and Pally were. At least they could look back with satisfaction on what they did, and the fans would appreciate it as well. In my case most of the fans would only remember an injury-prone little winger who never fulfilled the potential everyone said he had.

At least that's how I felt about things back then. With the MS slowly taking a firmer grip I became more estranged from the game of football than I could ever have imagined. I hadn't been near a football ground since the day I hobbled off the pitch in the colours of Mansfield Town. I had seen videos of my old games, of course, and I watched the football on television whenever I could. I still loved the game, but it was difficult coming to terms with the fact that I was no longer involved in any way. I missed it like mad, still do. But a funny thing happened to me at the age of 35. For some reason, a lot of the feelings of being cheated out of a career began to disappear. I knew that multiple sclerosis had stopped me playing the game and I had resented the fact that some of the best years of my life had been taken away from me because of the illness, but once I reached my mid-thirties a lot of the anger and frustration seemed to die down. It was as if I was raging only while I was still of an age to play top-class professional football; 35 and over was the sort of age when I would naturally have expected to stop playing anyway. If I was American, I suppose it was the sort of thing you could call 'closure'. I felt much more able to look forward rather than back all the time. I would always have my memories, my videos, my newspaper cuttings and a few medals and trophies as well, but the trick was to start enjoying them as good times. In this, naturally, Jenny had helped. 'When you start to feel down, have a look at them,' she had told me. 'They'll let you know how good you were and what a great life you've had.' As usual she was right, and I started to become much more realistic about myself and my new life, because that was how I had to begin looking at it.

*   *   *

At about the time when Alex was adding another trophy to his list of achievements, another manager in another part of Manchester was trying to work out how he could make sure he would have enough players to turn out a team for the new season.

Our former baby-sitter Alex Hartland, who was about thirteen when she had looked after Remi and Elisha when we first moved to Manchester, was now a young lady with a boyfriend called Paul Darbyshire. She still used to come round to see us sometimes, and Paul would come with her. He happened to mention one day that he and some of his mates played for a pub team called The Gatehouse, and asked me if I would be interested in getting involved by doing a bit of coaching and acting as their manager. The whole thing seemed to happen at the right time for me. I was just coming out of the really bad depression I'd had and was easing down on the drink. Had it been suggested a year earlier there was no way I would have considered it, but after joking about the idea with him and not really taking it seriously, it became clear that he thought it would be good for the team and that I would enjoy it. After all, it wasn't too serious; the only reason they played was because the guys he knew just liked to have an organised game every week.

I still wasn't really venturing out of the house, unless it was in the privacy of my car to do the school run with Thaila. I just didn't have the confidence. First of all my walking had really deteriorated, and so had the feeling in my right hand and foot. I was also still very much aware that people might stare at me as if I was some kind of freak. Not because of who I was or what I had been, but because I looked so strange when I was out on my own. At least, that was my perception. It wasn't the case at all, just another example of how low my self-esteem was. During the time I was drinking I would sometimes look at myself in the mirror to see what physical changes there had been. I looked the same until I started to move, and then I thought I looked strange. Nothing seemed co-ordinated, and if I looked like that when I was at home I could only imagine how I must look on the street. It was something that haunted me in a way, because I knew I had declined physically since the diagnosis. It was inevitable, and I had been told to expect it, but it still didn't really prepare me for the reality. To add to the problem, of course, I had then started drinking heavily, and while I felt better about myself when I had a glass in my hand, that soon wore off once the effects of the booze disappeared.

So getting involved in something like managing a pub team began to seem like a good idea, especially as far as Jenny was concerned, because she knew it would get me out of the house and hopefully back on the road to trying to rebuild my life. It might have only been a little thing, but she appreciated that it could lead on to other things. She had seen far worse cases than me work themselves back on to the road to recovery and knew from experience that it was really all about little building blocks. They might not look much on their own, but once they were pieced together they allowed people to reconstruct their shattered lives. Managing a pub team could start to help me manage my new life.

Paul, or 'Darbo' as he was known to the rest of the team, was a right-back and turned out to be a pretty good player; so too did a one-armed midfielder we had called Ant Morgan. I actually thought he had enough ability to make it in the professional game, and the team as a whole were a good bunch of guys who wanted to have fun and enjoyed their football. I organised a weekly training session for them and started to enjoy being in charge of a team. I also began to enjoy all the jokes and mickey-taking that went on. I'd missed it since packing in playing, and it was heartening to be involved again. The good thing was that it wasn't all about football. It was a social thing too, because after training and our matches on a Sunday we would all go back to the pub. The biggest problem I often had was getting a team together. A lot of the lads would have been out the night before a game and they sometimes had to cry off because of hangovers. It was a world away from what I'd been used to, and I loved every minute of it. Whenever I hear a manager on television moaning about his injury problems and being down to the bare bones of his squad, I often think back to when I was looking after The Gatehouse and we had to phone around on the morning of a match as we tried to get a team together. It's a scene that's repeated all over the country every week of the season, and it's part of the grassroots of the game. That didn't mean to say that all the teams were rubbish and just wanted a kickabout. Far from it: the matches were always very competitive, and you needed to be able to look after yourself out on the pitch.

I think a few people might have recognised me when I turned up to watch matches from the sidelines, but I never got into any conversations with people about what had happened to me and why I was no longer in the professional game. My brother Raymond came along and played for us a couple of times, and it was nice to have Remi in the side for a few matches as well. It was probably one of the few occasions we'd done something like that together, and it was also an opportunity for me to talk to him out of the house, because we would go back to the pub for a drink before going home.

I didn't think about it at the time, but those matches and all the training sessions and banter with the boys in the pub really helped me. I had a smile on my face again, and I was involved once more with the game I'd loved for so long. I was also interacting with people, real people who never gave the fact that I had MS a second thought. I was just Danny, the guy who managed them and knew a bit about football. I also started to receive visitors again because a few of the lads would come over to the house sometimes. That helped me as well. I still hadn't snapped out of my gloom completely – I would still have a go at Jenny and the kids from time to time, my mood still swinging from being nice one moment to being nasty the next depending on what sort of day I'd had – but I was getting there.

Typically, one of the bad moments involved me having a really terrible row with Remi. He had been out with some of his friends and then decided to sit up watching television. I told him to go to bed, and I started shouting at him before pushing him. Remi pushed me back, and not only was he bigger than me, I was also unable to balance properly. It would have looked comical had anyone been watching, but it's only effect on me was to make me angrier, and I swung at him with my fist. It wasn't a good thing to do, and I could see in his eyes that Remi was wondering what the hell had happened to me. The truth was I was still coming to terms with my life and what it had become. I'd had a bad day that day, with constant pain in my back. I was at a low point, and Remi caught the full force of it. It wasn't the right thing to do and I'm not proud of it, but although there were still moments like those, at least I was aware that I had to learn to deal with them in a different way.

The truth was, I had started to make progress. I was beginning to get my life together, though I knew that the process might be both physically and mentally painful.

CHAPTER SEVENTEEN

ONE IN A MILLION

Over the eighteen months after my 35th birthday in January 1999, which when I look back I think of as the point at which I began to make progress, the picture of what my life would be like became clearer for me, and the person who did so much to help me see that picture was Jenny. She was the one who saw at first hand how the MS affected me, how it tortured me in body and in mind. And she was the one who saw past my self-centred behaviour and never stopped believing that I loved her.

I've mentioned the many times my selfish actions meant that I only looked after myself and at the same time neglected her. I'd treated her badly in the past, right from the time when we were both kids and I was an apprentice at Southampton. Football is a great game, and being a professional is a great career, but it does sometimes mean that players are given the licence to carry on being schoolboys long after they have started work and are earning the sort of money most men in the street can only dream of. If you want to, you can carry on doing the sort of things you have always done and put off growing up. I'm not saying all footballers are like that, but I think I certainly was. How else can I explain the fact that I had Jenny and Remi living in London while I lived the single life in Southampton? Why did I think nothing of going out with my mates to nightclubs after matches while Jen stayed at home? And how could I ever have gone off with friends a couple of days after Jenny had a miscarriage and was sobbing at home in our bedroom? There was no excuse for my behaviour, but I think Jen knew me well enough to realise that there was no spite or malice in what I did. I was stupid and immature; she realised that I never meant to upset her. There were plenty of times when she rightly read the riot act to me, but at the same time she knew I loved her and had done so from the very first day we went out together.

There was a mutual attraction there from the start, although I've never really been able to fathom exactly what she saw in me. There was certainly no shortage of boys who wanted to go out with her, and I think she did see a few of them when we had that period when I was in Southampton and she was still in London. We were teenagers then, and it's amazing that we both decided we would stay together and see each other every two or three weeks. I often think things like that prove that we were meant to be together. We could so easily have broken up and gone our separate ways. Although we did see other people, there was a kind of unspoken agreement that we would remain together as boyfriend and girlfriend. Nobody was forcing us, it was just something we wanted, and we stuck to it.

Having her and Remi with me in Southampton should have settled me down more – certainly that was what Lawrie McMenemy must have been hoping when he spoke to the two of us and arranged for somewhere for us to stay – but I continued to act like the schoolboy I still was at heart. I wasn't a bad person, but I was thoughtless when it came to Jenny, and it amazes me that she didn't walk out. If she had been the sort of person who is afraid to say what she thinks I might have understood it more, but Jen is more than capable of giving as good as she gets, and then a bit more on top. There were quite a few times when we had rows and I left the house thinking that when I got back she might be gone for good, but it never happened, and the bond that had been there from the start was probably the reason it didn't. We weren't just boyfriend and girlfriend, or man and wife, we were best mates.

To a large extent I have always relied on her and she has always been there for me. A lot of the time I know I took her for granted, but I always loved her, and we'd had some great times as a couple and as a family with the kids. But it was always basically a case of me getting on with my life as a footballer and leaving everything else for her to sort out. With the onset of my multiple sclerosis, her best qualities – kindness, caring, understanding – were tested to the limit. How she coped with what she went through, or more precisely what I put her through, I shall never know. The phrase may sound corny, but as far as I'm concerned she really is one in a million. I simply could not have coped without her, and neither could the children. At a time when I was hit by MS and then went missing mentally because of depression and booze, she was the one who held the family together. Not just on an emotional level but on a very practical one as well. Without her working virtually around the clock on some occasions we wouldn't have survived financially, and to this day it is her salary that keeps us afloat.

I might have been the one with the illness, but Jenny has been a sufferer as well. I know that during the worst days, when I was moping around the house and drinking, she was worried sick by what she saw. At one stage she told me bluntly that she thought I was waiting to die because of what I was doing to myself. She had to go off to work and cope with the kids while her husband sank lower and lower into depression. She knew I was using the drink as a crutch and must have gone through all sorts of anxieties wondering if I would ever come to my senses. When I finally began to emerge from the dark tunnel I'd been content to use as a hiding place from the real world, Jenny knew I would need all the help and support she could give me to make sure I didn't return to my bad old ways. My birthday, Thaila, The Gatehouse team – they were all little building blocks which she knew I could use to help me re-design my life. I needed reassurance that I had a future, no matter how different it might be, and Jenny provided it.

I also needed to reinforce the fact that my boozing had to stay in the past, and one day I got help in that direction from an unexpected source. The group of mates I used to go out with on a regular basis when I was in Southampton were people I'd known for most of my life. They were old school friends, or people who had lived near me in Deptford, and we had grown up together. When I became a footballer they were delighted for me because they knew how much I had wanted to succeed in the professional game. They didn't treat me any differently when I started to do well and I always felt comfortable in their company. They used to love coming down for weekends and going out drinking in clubs with me, and even when we moved north to Manchester they would still visit, although the trips weren't as frequent because of the distance.

One of my mates, Ted, used to love coming to Manchester as much as he enjoyed travelling down for weekends to Southampton. On one of his visits he met a girl and decided he would move up from the south and set up home with her. It wasn't too long after this that I found out about my MS and began to discourage all of my old friends from visiting. As I said, I just didn't want people around, and after the falling-over incident outside the Manchester nightclub I didn't want to be seen out with a group of blokes any more either. As a consequence I stopped seeing people like Ted for quite a while, and we lost contact. But one day, completely out of the blue, he turned up at our house, and when I opened the front door both Jenny and I had to do a double-take. Ted had always been a slim, fit, healthy-looking guy, but the figure standing in front of us that day looked podgy and bloated. It was Ted's head all right, but it looked as though it had been put on a different body. Even his face looked puffy. It was obvious he'd had a pretty rough time. We found out from talking to him that he'd split up with his girlfriend some time ago, had had a bad time with his job, and had fallen into a depression. Like me, he had hit the bottle, but in a bigger way, drinking vodka and turning himself into a virtual alcoholic. If I needed a warning sign of what might happen to me if I carried on drinking, Ted provided it for me that day.

It was another building block, and I took notice of it. So did Jenny. I think she began to see during this period that I was showing signs of wanting to come to terms with my life after being unwilling to do so ever since I had been diagnosed, and she knew that she needed to seize the opportunity. It must have been a relief for her to see me slowly coming out of the depression that had engulfed me, even if it was a gradual thing interrupted occasionally by relapses when I would start to feel sorry for myself again. The good thing was that the solitary drinking began to stop and my existence during the daytime became much more normal. Instead of reaching for the brandy bottle after taking Thaila to school, I was reaching for the cornflakes again. I didn't feel the need to sit in front of the television and drink, and I actually started to do some of the little jobs around the house that Jenny gave me before she went off to work. First time round she'd done this in an attempt to switch my focus away from the drinking; now she was doing it to give my day some sort of structure. She knew that the more I did the quicker the time would go, and I wouldn't get the chance to sit around and think.

Although I'd dabbled in cooking before, it had never been that serious, but I suddenly started to get interested in it. I watched the cooking programmes on television and then tried to recreate the dishes for Jenny and the kids. Once she saw that I was serious about it all, Jen went out and bought me some cookbooks, and I would spend quite a bit of time preparing a meal and trying it out on her. Alongside the cooking, Jen would also ask me to make phone calls for her – which may not sound like a big deal, but I had become so fed up at one stage that I didn't like talking to people on the phone. I tried to tidy up the house and clean it as well, but that sometimes had disastrous consequences, because my walking had deteriorated and so had my ability to grip anything in my right hand. If I tried to do something as simple as use a duster, for instance, it would keep falling out of my hand; if I was vacuuming, as I walked across the room I would often hit or trip over something and end up on the floor. Jenny would also put clothes on for a wash before she went out of the house in the morning; all I had to do was get them out of the machine and put them in the dryer, but more often than not I'd get myself into trouble trying to pick things up and bend over at the same time.

It may sound incredible to people who have no idea of the effects of MS, but the fact is that one of the worst things about the disease isn't the pain and discomfort, it's the way it either stops you doing very ordinary things or makes it extremely difficult for you to cope with them. Jenny appreciated this, and once again her work with the NHS must have come in useful. She knew how people with disabilities sometimes struggled to cope with their lives, and she knew how those lives had to be adapted to help them cope. One of the things Jen decided to do at home was remove any ornaments that were on or close to the floor, so that I didn't bash into them if I fell over. I once went to bed without realising that I had blood oozing out of a gash on my back. When Jenny saw it she naturally asked what had happened. I didn't have a clue at first, but then I remembered that an hour or so earlier I had fallen over on to an ornament near the fire. Sure enough, when Jen went downstairs to investigate the broken object was all over the place, and so was some of my blood.

Doing jobs around the house was one thing, but Jenny knew the real test was trying to convince me to start going out more. I still did the school runs and I'd got a lot more self-confidence after managing The Gatehouse pub team. Mixing with people in a social context after training and matches had really been useful, but I was still self-conscious enough not to want to be seen out that often, and Jenny knew it was another problem I had to overcome if I wanted to move on. One day she asked me if I would go with her to do the weekly supermarket shopping, and although I was reluctant, I eventually agreed to go. We drove off to Tesco, but once we got there my bottle went a bit and instead of getting out and going into the store I stayed in the car and read a newspaper. This happened on two or three occasions: every time at the last minute I would panic at the thought of trying to walk about in such a crowded place in front of so many people.

But one day that changed. Jenny asked me to go into the supermarket and I said yes. I honestly don't know what the trigger was, I just finally decided I would follow her in. I went up and down every aisle, and then waited at the check-out next to her as she struggled to pack everything into plastic bags. I didn't attempt to help because I knew that if I picked anything up with my right hand the likelihood was that I would drop it, so I let Jen get on with it. She just seemed happy that I'd managed to take another step forward and smiled as I stood there watching her. But then she suddenly stopped. 'Dan,' she said, 'I know you can't use your right hand, but there's nothing wrong with that left one, so start packing some stuff with it!' We both burst out laughing, mainly because we knew there had been a massive breakthrough. People had seen me, of course, but I don't really think they paid any attention. I just looked like a little black guy who walked with a limp. Nobody pointed or made comments, and nobody really recognised me. If they did they didn't come up and pester me or ask questions about what had happened. Those things were always in the back of my mind when I became ill, and it was the main reason for me not wanting to go out or meet people. I had felt awkward and embarrassed, which of course was stupid, so that trip to Tesco really did help me, and once again it was Jenny who had encouraged and guided me further along the road to a new life.

I'm sure I wasn't the first or last person with MS or another disability who has felt that way. I know there are other people out there who have got MS and are suffering in worse ways, but I'm sure each one of us has gone through similar emotions, with the 'Why me?' question at the top of the list. That's what it can do. It not only has some bad physical effects, it can mentally change you and the way you look at the rest of the world. If you are not strong enough and don't have the right people around you, it can be a nightmare. I was lucky and blessed to have Jenny. She took the time and the trouble to coax me out of the gloom and give me hope. The more I think about what has happened since that first diagnosis, the more I realise just how fortunate I have been. When you first learn that you have the illness it seems as though you are totally on your own. You feel like an isolated figure. It took me a long time to come to terms with the fact that it wasn't like that, and also to realise what an idiot I had been to try to keep Jenny at arm's length for so long.

When things started to get better between us and I began to open up and talk to her about the way I felt and the fears I had, it was like a weight being lifted from my shoulders. She had always wanted to help and be there for me – as far as she was concerned it wasn't just about me having a problem, it was about us – and once we did start to talk the tears seemed to flow just as quickly as the words came out of our mouths. We had a lot of catching up to do on the emotional front, and the reason for that was me. I was the one who had taken the decision not to communicate, and instead to look inwards. I wasn't prepared to open up to Jenny or anyone else, and because of that I suffered, and she suffered along with me. But she always had faith that I would come through it all, that in the end she would be left with the Danny she always believed was in there somewhere.

After all the shit I had put her and the children through, I began to feel that I had something to look forward to. I wasn't exactly sure what it was, and I knew that physically I was never going to be the same man I had been, but I was certain that I'd come through the really bad times and was heading in the right direction.

CHAPTER EIGHTEEN

PANIC IN THE SHEETS

I had just woken up after a decent night's sleep and was lying in bed taking it easy before preparing myself for the start of another day. Jenny put her arm across and touched me on the shoulder, and suddenly I was experiencing the most frightening few seconds of my life.

My entire body locked up. Arms, hands, legs, feet. I found myself in the foetal position with my fingers curled and rigid. I was in complete panic, and for the short period it lasted I seriously thought my body was going to stay that way. I couldn't move any of my limbs, and the only thing I could do was scream out in pain. It must have been frightening for Jenny as well because it was the first time anything like that had happened. She just stared at me open-mouthed. Then, just as rapidly as it had come, the spasm subsided and disappeared, leaving me gasping for air in a pool of my own sweat.

That first spasm occurred soon after I had been diagnosed with MS, and in the years that followed I grew used to them. Although the pain and experience of having one of the attacks is still horrible, I have learnt to cope. I know it will go away eventually and my muscles and body will unwind and relax. I know it will only last a matter of seconds as well, but it doesn't stop it from being one of the worst effects of the illness. I get a spasm just about every day, even though they are now much more under control than they used to be. I take a drug called Tizanidine which helps to keep the ferocity of them in check, but they still occur, and I know I will experience them for the rest of my life. I also experience relapses about four times a year when I'm not able to get out of bed for three days because my body is just too tired and locked up to do anything other than rest. I can even tell when one of the attacks is on the way because I always fall over more just before I have one. I also fall over just after a spasm has gone. Although you can never fully get over the fact that your body is going to react like that on a regular basis, I've found that I am now prepared for them. Not only that, Jen and I can joke about the situation as well. She'll sometimes threaten to touch me if I'm getting on her nerves, knowing that something as innocuous as that can sometimes trigger an attack.

When the attack comes, all my muscles stiffen up. It's a bit like having cramp in every part of your body, and that's why it hurts so much. I remember getting cramp during the first FA Cup final match with Palace, and that hurt. I managed to run it off and get on with playing, but with the spasms there is no way you can do anything except stay locked up in one position and wait for it to subside. Jenny has timed them, and we know they only last for a few seconds, but it feels like ages when it's actually happening and it seems as though it's never going to end.

Although spasms are one of the worst aspects of my MS, with Jenny's help, as I said, I began to discover ways of dealing with some of the other effects. I couldn't have had anyone better than Jenny to help me; because of her and the children I knew there was a real purpose to my life after all. There were still times when I was feeling under the weather and I took it out on her or the kids, though. My relationship with Remi was still far from perfect. We had rows, sometimes they got ugly, and sometimes Jenny had to step in between us. My relationship with Elisha seemed to be better, even though I know I hadn't been there for her either when she was young. Thaila, of course, I was very close to. It was no coincidence that he had been the only one of our children I had been around for. The time we spent together was bound to bond us, and although I was delighted it had, I was also sad and full of regret that it couldn't have been like that with Remi and Elisha. At least with Elisha I had a bit of a second chance, because she was still young enough to be around for a few years after I began to improve mentally, and I hope that more recently I have been a better dad to her than I was in the first part of her life. At least she knew where to find me because

I couldn't go too far and I wasn't about to go for long nights out with my mates!

Mind you, I did try another night out with the boys when Paul Ince asked me over to Liverpool near Christmas time in 1998. I honestly didn't fancy going, and if it had been anyone other than Incy I would have made an excuse and not bothered. But he'd been a good friend to me and we'd kept in touch, even when he and Claire were in Italy following his transfer to Inter Milan. Liverpool had paid £4.2 million to bring him back to England, and he insisted that I come and have a good time out on the town with him and the rest of the Liverpool boys. He told me they all wanted me to go along and that I would enjoy it. Jenny was keen for me to go as well. The fact that there might be a few drinks involved didn't bother her: she seemed to know that by that time I was beginning to get over the worst of my brandy phase and realised that I wasn't likely to relapse after one night out.

So I headed off for the short trip to Liverpool and met up with Paul and the rest of the lads. They were all in good spirits, as you might expect for a players' night out, and it wasn't long before we were heading to a club. But while they were all off and moving around the place, I had to grab a seat. I soon started to feel out of it. Everyone was really friendly and made me feel welcome, but as much as I wanted to be part of the group and to remember what it was like to be out with a load of footballers, I couldn't help feeling isolated. Not because of them, because of me. I wanted to be like them and join in everything they were doing, but I physically wasn't able to do it. To cap the whole night the inevitable finally happened: I lost my balance, took a tumble and hit the floor. I remember Micky Thomas rushing over to help me up, and I did my usual by waving him away and saying I would be all right, but the truth was I was far from all right. I was a disabled man suffering from the effects of MS trying to have a night out with a group of super-fit professional footballers, and I felt and looked out of place. It was one of those bad times that occurred along the way. Happily, though I've suffered that sort of setback on more than one occasion, I've managed to overcome them and carry on.

Walking became progressively harder for me. Eventually it seemed as though the only way I could move forward was by dragging my right foot along. Jenny suggested I use a cane, but I was too proud and stubborn to take her advice. I continued to take my chances without one, and of course I paid the price several times. The funny thing is that you almost get used to finding yourself flat on your arse. If I'd gone over as spectacularly as that when I was playing football I'm sure I would have earned so many more penalties in my career than I did!

Jenny and I had to basically map out each day of my life. Obviously if I was at home things were a lot easier, because the house was familiar territory, and although I still went for a tumble every now and then it was better if it happened there rather than out on the street. Because multiple sclerosis affects the muscles, it means that your body just doesn't function as well as it used to. The most obvious sign of that with me was my limp and the fact that I really couldn't use or grip with my right hand. But there were other basic things like going to the toilet that sometimes had to be planned with military precision. When I wanted to have a pee I had to be able to go straight away; there was no way I could hold myself and wait to get to a toilet. If I needed to wee, it happened right there and then. I've lost count of the times I've had accidents because I simply haven't had time to make it to the toilet. It's a bit of a double whammy: I need to go instantly, but when I do try to get to a toilet my limp means it will take me longer than it would an able-bodied person. Because of that, when I go out anywhere one of my first thoughts is to find out where the toilet is. If I'm in a restaurant or out shopping with Jenny, we have to work out where they are and how long it will take me to get to them. If I can, I will always sit near a toilet. Even if we go out to someone's house, one of the first questions will be to ask them where their bathroom is.

You just become so much more aware of your body and your life. Physically, every minute of every day I know I will have to deal with what MS has done to me. It's not like a cold or a bad case of the flu, which will eventually go away. I know my MS won't. I also know that it won't get any better. Hopefully it won't get any worse than it is at the moment either, but I realise that it could, and if it does I'll have to deal with it. I feel better equipped to do that now, and the reason for that is Jenny, who has helped me put in all the groundwork to cope with my new life. It was a case of being more patient and less self-conscious as well. Once upon a time I would keep everyone at arm's length and insist that I didn't need help, which was really stupid. The one thing you really have to recognise early on is that the more help you can get the better. I remember once sitting at home with Jenny and one of her friends having a drink. I got up to walk across the room and managed to fall over, spilling my drink everywhere and landing on my back. Jen and her mate rushed over to help me get up, but I shouted at them to go away and let me pull myself up. But have you ever tried to get up from the floor using just one leg? It's virtually impossible, especially because at the time my back happened to feel as though there was a steel rod running from the top to the bottom and I had no flexibility at all. 'Dan,' Jenny said as she looked down at me scrabbling around on the floor, 'let us pick you up, otherwise we'll give you a wedgie for your trouble as well!' Not for the first time she was right, and I had to swallow my pride and let the two girls pick me up from the floor. The simple fact is that if you are not prepared to do things like that then your life will be an awful lot worse. You have to take every opportunity to ease the pain and the sheer inconvenience of having MS.

There is, of course, a more controversial method of achieving this end. I have a constant feeling of pins and needles in my right hand and right foot, as well as the back pain that has become part of my everyday existence. Sometimes the pain gets so bad that all the drugs prescribed by the doctors just don't seem to work. Jenny and I started to read about the illness once I had started to come to terms with it. We discovered that a lot had been written about what can actually alleviate the pain sufferers get, and one of the things which seemed to help some people was cannabis.

I had only ever tried the stuff once in my life, during the celebrations after United's European Cup Winners' Cup win in 1991, and hadn't particularly enjoyed it, but I felt I had to try something to ease the constant pain I was experiencing. Until you have pain with you twenty-four hours a day it is impossible to understand how desperate you become for some relief from it. The cannabis did that for me, and I know it has done the same for lots of MS sufferers all over the world. I'm not advocating it for everyone, but I know it worked for me. I think it helped to relax me, and my muscles and body responded in a similar way. I've smoked the stuff several times for the same reason, even though I can't stand things like cigarettes. The first time I tried it I had to force myself to inhale because it was a weird feeling for me to be doing something like that. The only drug that hadn't been prescribed that I'd ever gone near before that was alcohol of course, and although the brandy did have a relaxing effect it was never the same as cannabis. I honestly think the authorities and medical people ought to look into whether it can have a positive effect for some people who have MS.

But one of the things pills and such measures cannot do is help you cope mentally. One of the reasons why I had found the process of being positive about life again so difficult was that not only did I have the illness, I had also had to suffer quite a long period of not knowing about it. Of course, that is the same for most people who eventually find out that they have MS, but in quite a lot of those cases they might be in jobs where it is possible for them to return to work in some form or another. In my case that simply wasn't possible. I was a footballer; if I couldn't play football any more my career was over. There was no support network that there might have been in other jobs. Perhaps if I had worked in a bank, for instance, I could have gone back and done some sort of job and continued to interact with work colleagues. But that all stopped for me the moment I left the game. Don't get me wrong, I know how lucky I am ever to have been a professional footballer and I will always be grateful that I was, and also that I earned such a good living from it. But it certainly made it harder to accept what had happened to me. When you have taken being able to run a hundred yards in a matter of seconds for granted, it comes as a real shock to the system to find that you will only ever be able to shuffle along for the rest of your life.

Although apart from The Gatehouse pub team I hadn't really been involved in football since walking away from that Mansfield match, I still loved the game and would always watch any match that was on the television. I hadn't gone to many games since retiring, but I'd seen Rodney playing for Glasgow Rangers and Raymond turning out for Stoke City. Both of them had moved on from Leeds, and I was happy to see the two of them still playing and enjoying their football. But apart from those matches my actual contact with the professional game was pretty minimal. Not too many people in the game even knew what had happened to me.

Ambrose Mendy, who had acted as an agent for me when I went down to speak to Southampton in 1993, is someone you might politely describe as 'a bit of a character'. He's had a chequered career – at the top one moment and representing sports stars, behind bars the next for various misdemeanours. He was always very good to me, though, and was always ready to help if he could. One day towards the end of 1999 he phoned me to ask what I thought about having a benefit match staged for me by Manchester United. I have to admit that the thought had never entered my head, particularly as I'd left the club having failed to fulfil my potential. But Ambrose seemed to think something could be done, and when I put the phone down I had to admit that I felt excited by the prospect. I still watched as many of United's matches as I could, and seeing them lift the Champions League title that night in May 1999 had been fantastic. I tried not to get too carried away with the thought of something happening for me, but it was difficult not to start thinking about the possibility. Even if nothing came of it, I liked the idea of maybe seeing some of the people I had once known and catching up on old times.

Once upon a time I would have been horrified at the thought of being seen again at Old Trafford looking the way I did, but that wasn't the case any more. All the hard work Jenny had done with me was paying off. I was starting to act and feel more normal. I no longer felt the need to hide away and not let anyone know where I was or what had happened to me. If people wanted to ask me about my MS, I would give them an answer. I had got over the feelings of resentment at the loss of my career. I had started to build a new life, and despite all the difficulties I was determined to make it work for me. If nothing else, I owed it to Jenny and the children to make sure that happened.

CHAPTER NINETEEN

GAME ON

In fact, the possibility of having a game staged for my benefit had a really positive effect on me. I had already started to make steady progress of course, but the idea of having football back in my life again, and with a team like Manchester United involved, gave me another massive boost.

Talks soon started, the idea to try to stage a match between United and Southampton. I took a back seat in all the discussions. First of all I didn't really think it was right that I should push myself forward, and secondly, I preferred to leave it to people who knew what they were doing. United seemed very receptive to the idea, and it became clear that they genuinely wanted to try to do something for me. Martin Edwards was the chairman when I signed for the club back in 1989, and it was good to know that he still thought enough of me to get United involved in the project. The trouble was, they were just too busy. By this time Manchester United were just about the biggest thing in British football, and they also had fans all around the world. Not only did they have commitments in all the domestic competitions, they were also heavily involved in Europe, and when it came to free dates their calendar had been mapped out far in advance. I know they wanted to do something, they just weren't able to find a time and date when a game could be staged. It was disappointing, but it simply couldn't be helped. Still, once it was clear they wouldn't be able to host a game, Martin Edwards and United did something which showed just how big they were, not in the sense of their size as a club but in the way they went about things.

I have already mentioned that although I earned very good money during my career, it was by no means enough for me to sit back in the lap of luxury once I had to retire. We used a lot of our savings to start up our sandwich business, and then to help supplement the money Jenny earned from her jobs. We also spent some money on legal fees for a couple of years when we began an action for damages against Birmingham for what I believed was their failure to investigate the underlying cause of my injury problems. The idea for believing there might be grounds for a claim came from Ambrose Mendy, and he put us in touch with a firm of London solicitors who started to look into the situation. We spent thousands of pounds on the research and preparation of a case – the lawyers obtained as much medical evidence as they could, including records from Southampton, Manchester United, Birmingham and Wycombe, and also got opinions from internationally renowned physiotherapists and other medical experts – but eventually we were advised to drop it because it was thought we didn't have a strong enough chance of winning, and we could end up losing even more money. There was my PFA pension, which was a help, but although we were never skint, it's fair to say that the Wallace household was far from being flush with cash. But then, after United realised they wouldn't be able to host a benefit match for me, Martin Edwards arranged for the club to give me a cheque for £30,000 to help with my finances and to go towards medical bills. It was a wonderful gesture, and I have to admit that the money came in very handy at the time.

The investigation of the possibility of having a game at Old Trafford generated some publicity, and that meant that people began to learn about the fact that I had multiple sclerosis. It was another step in the right direction for me, because I found that I was happier to talk about my condition than I thought I would be. If an ex-footballer like me could raise awareness of the illness, then that was fine. I'm sure there are a lot of sufferers out there who never really think that MS will touch people like sportsmen and sportswomen. Of course it does, and even if you've never played at the highest level there are plenty of people who were extremely active and who enjoyed their sport before being struck down with the condition. Most football clubs have a lot of disabled supporters, and the good thing nowadays is that there is much more awareness of disability and what it means. In my playing days you might get one or two people sitting in wheelchairs at one end of the ground or at the side of the pitch, but it was almost as if it was a token effort. These days there are special sections around the ground, and the stadiums themselves are much more user-friendly for disabled supporters.

Manchester United have a disabled supporters' club, and it was through them that I got an unexpected call one day. It came from a guy called Mick Wood, a disabled Newcastle supporter who had found out about me having MS. He was a sufferer as well, and after chatting on the phone it was clear that we had a lot in common. It was also good to talk football with him, and since that day Mick and I have stayed in contact. I've met up with him as well. Talking to him was good for me, and I realised that it was probably the first time I had spoken to a fellow sufferer, which was crazy. It's good to talk, as they say, and I knew that I hadn't really done enough of it. Not being afraid to speak up and talk openly about MS was therapeutic for me, and I started to do more of it.

Once again it was Jenny who got me started on the right road: she took me along to a ten-week counselling course on which she had enrolled to help with her NHS work. There were about a dozen people there each of whom had to stand up and talk about themselves before we even got going. The idea was to give a real insight into what you were about as a person and the sort of life you had. Now, I've never felt comfortable having to stand up in a group and talk. In fact, I used to hate doing things like television interviews when I was playing because I was a naturally shy person. I used to carry a handkerchief in my pocket on all occasions just so that I could wipe my forehead because I used to sweat so much. But those sessions were really useful to me. Even if I didn't attend all of them, Jen knew that the overall effect would be a positive one, and she was right.

By this time things were looking a lot better for me. I was happy to be living my life in a better frame of mind, and my relationship with Jenny had just gone from strength to strength. I had gone through something which was quite literally life-changing when I found out I had MS, and I had come to realise that without Jenny's love and devotion I simply would not have had a life. For most people, getting the illness feels like the worst thing that can ever happen to them, but in my case, out of it all came one of the best things ever to happen to me: Jenny and I became closer. We still had the odd cross word, just like any other married couple, but any bad situation tended to get defused pretty quickly, and it was normally Jenny's sense of humour that did that. We talked a lot, and we talked about everything. She was there for me all the time. There was nothing she wouldn't do for me, including things like bed baths when I just felt too exhausted to get up. Sometimes that feeling could last for two or three days. She was the one who took care of me, the house, the family, and the small matter of going out to work to earn some money. Our relationship became very honest and very open, and it has stayed that way to this day. I would be totally lost without her, and she knows it. I'm just glad that I happened to be married to someone who could give so much and stay so happy. Throughout all that went on, Jenny was the one who tried to keep a smile on her face, even though it must have been incredibly difficult for her. She has more strength and character than I ever will, and there isn't a day that goes by now without me thanking God that she is with me.

Towards the end of 2002, the subject of a benefit match in my honour cropped up again. This time it was George Lawrence who came up with the idea – a testimonial at Southampton. George had been a good friend of mine during our time at Southampton, and when he went off to play for teams like Oxford, Millwall and Portsmouth we kept in touch, but it was probably an indication of just how low I was feeling after being diagnosed that I didn't even bother telling him I had the illness and didn't make the effort to keep in touch. It was George who eventually spoke to me and finally got the story of what had been happening to me. Since then we had talked occasionally on the phone, and he began to help me do some bits and pieces that were connected to football. After finishing his playing career, George had become a football agent, and he also turned out for The Saints veterans' team. He had maintained a far closer connection with the club than I had and often saw some of the lads we both used to play alongside when we were all at Southampton.

Having had the experience of the attempt at organising something with United, I have to say that I didn't raise my hopes too high. Still, somehow the fact that it was Southampton seemed to make me feel it was more likely. George got hold of Matt Le Tissier and put the proposal to him. Suddenly, within the space of a few months, the whole idea seemed to take off and it really did look as though the game would be on. George and Matt formed a committee, and we secured the co-operation of Southampton chairman Rupert Lowe and the club for a game to be staged in May 2004. The idea was to have a Southampton team playing against an all-star side which would be made up of various players I'd known during my career, and the team was going to be managed by Lawrie McMenemy. George was the driving force behind the venture, and once I knew that it was definitely going to happen I have to admit that it gave me a huge mental lift. For the next year and more leading up to the testimonial my life had a real sense of purpose and direction, mainly because of all the planning and publicity that had to be done. I realised I had missed being out of the limelight, and for a brief time I didn't mind being back in it. I also liked having a connection with Southampton again. The club had always been like a second family for me. There was a very real sense of coming home.

By this time the club had moved from The Dell and played their football at the brand new St Mary's Stadium. A couple of weeks before my game was due to be played I was invited down to watch Southampton play in a Premiership match against Bolton. It was also an opportunity for me to do some publicity with the media, letting everyone know about my testimonial. The local television station, Meridian, suggested I do an interview with them on the pitch a couple of hours before the game started. The stadium was empty apart from a group of stewards who were getting their pre-match briefing on the far side of the ground. The TV people wanted me to walk along the pitch. I was using a cane by then, but it was still a bit of a problem, and I must have looked as though I was hobbling rather than walking. Just as I started to move, I heard some cheers and clapping. I looked across the pitch and saw the stewards. They were all standing up and cheering. At first I thought all the noise was for someone else, but then I realised it was for me. Now I really knew I was home.

The reception I got during the match from the crowd was overwhelming. As I stood on the pitch and waved to the fans, I must admit that I had a tear in my eye. I'm sure a lot of those supporters had never seen me play, but they still knew about me, and that meant an awful lot. And those fans who had seen me obviously must have thought I'd done a decent job for the club while I was there. It meant the world to me, as did the actual testimonial. In fact, that night was one of the best and most emotional of my life. As well as all the Southampton boys who gave up their time to play, the All-Star side's squad featured Mark Dennis, Steve Baker, Paul Ince, Cyrille Regis, Luther Blissett, Jimmy Case, John Barnes, Clayton Blackmore, Franny Benali, Dennis Rofe, Steve Williams, Mickey Adams, Kevin Moore, Mark Wright, Nick Holmes, Ian Baird, Denis Irwin, Kevin Bond, Dave Beasant, Tim Flowers, Jean Tigana, Martin Chivers, Viv Anderson, Steve Moran, Russell Osman, Gordon Strachan and Graham Baker, alongside Matt, George, Remi and my brothers Raymond and Rodney. My half brother Paul was also there to see the game and the only sad note was that my dad wasn't there to witness it. He had really been looking forward to the game but tragically died two months earlier as he battled against a heart problem. We thought for a while that Incy wasn't going to turn up, but he arrived late and put in a great performance. He was still playing full-time for Wolves so he was as fit as anyone on the pitch. Matt Le Tissier showed once again that he is one of the best players this country has ever produced, with all the skill, flair and touches the Southampton fans had come to know over the years on display. It was great to see my two brothers out there as well. Rodney helped the All-Stars get back in the game after David Prutton had scored for

Southampton. Rod was brought down in the area and it was just like old times for the two of them as Matt made no mistake from the spot. Big Cyrille Regis also got on the scoresheet for the All-Stars with the sort of well-taken goal he had made his name with, and Brett Ormerod netted for Saints as honours ended even at 2–2.

I was thrilled that all those players had made the effort to be there and make it a special occasion. It was great to see them all again, and to catch up with all the stories of what had been happening to them. Big Lawrie enjoyed being in charge too. Just for old times' sake, he even let me call him by his Christian name without giving me a clip around the ear, as he had done at Old Trafford on my debut all those years ago. It really was a magical night for me, and a reminder that no matter what had happened I was still a very fortunate person.

CHAPTER TWENTY

MAN WITH A PLAN

Around 14,000 people turned out for that benefit match at St Mary's, and after various bits and pieces had been deducted from the takings, I was given a cheque for £110,000. Once again I was grateful for the money, and it has helped us over the last couple of years with our finances. I was surprised just how much of the overall money seemed to go on incidental costs, but really, I don't want to sound ungrateful. In fact, I want to thank each and every one of those supporters who made the effort to come along that night, not to mention the players and other people behind the scenes who made it such a lovely occasion for me. People really rallied round for me, and it made me realise how terrific football people can be, and how lucky I was. Alan Ball was one of the former players who had agreed to play in the testimonial for me, but in the end he had to pull out because his wife died shortly before the match was played. It was typical of Bally that even at a terrible time like that for him he still insisted on sending his son along to play in the game for me.

Tragedy strikes all sorts of people in all sorts of ways every day. I might have MS, but I also have a life, and I plan to make the most of it. The testimonial was a big part of me being able to say that. It was so heartening to know that I hadn't been forgotten by the fans, that there was so much love and warmth out there for me. For a couple of years after being diagnosed with multiple sclerosis I wasted my life, filling it with drink and depression. I was so fortunate to have Jenny to lead me in the right direction and help rebuild things. She gave me the purpose I needed and taught me that I had to get on with things in the best way I could, just as anyone else has to. Within the space of about two years I went from playing at Old Trafford with Manchester United to having a trial with Mansfield. After the diagnosis of multiple sclerosis my life hit rock bottom, but in time I came to realise it wasn't the end of the world, it was just a different kind of world. With the help and love of my wife and family I've learned to cope with that world and understand that it still offers me all sorts of opportunities. I know that there are people out there right now who have MS and feel alone, angry and in pain. Like I did, they probably think nobody else understands how they feel or what is going on in their lives, but that is never the case. There really is always someone else worse off than you, and the most important thing is to appreciate exactly what you do have and then build on it.

After wasting so much time wallowing in self-pity, I now know that being positive about my condition is as important as all the medication I have to take. Multiple sclerosis is a terrible, debilitating illness that can change lives for ever, but the important thing is to meet it head on and not allow yourself to be beaten by it. Even today I sometimes find it difficult to come to terms with the reality of my life, but trying to hide away from it is worse. I finally gave in to common sense a few years ago and started using a cane to help me walk. I should have been using it years earlier, but stubbornness and pride stopped me. Stupid, I know, but it was another lesson I had to learn the hard way. Last summer we went to Alton Towers with some friends and their kids. If I had tried to walk around the place it would have taken ages, so instead I swallowed my pride and opted for a wheelchair. As an added bonus we all got taken to the front of the line for every ride we went on!

It is so important to be sensible enough to keep on adapting the way I live and do things. If, for instance, sometimes using a wheelchair makes it easier for me and those around me, then I will use one. It is all part of dealing with my illness and being honest to myself about it. Years ago it came as a bit of a shock when I could no longer put a pair of trousers on without falling over, but I learnt to sit down and do it slowly. At first it made me feel depressed – another simple thing I could no longer do – but after a time you come to terms with the problem and it is just another part of your life which has to be re-designed. The main thing is to move forward and not lose sight of the bigger picture.

I feel there is more of a plan to my life now than there probably ever has been, certainly since first learning that I had MS. I have, for instance, set up my own foundation, the Danny Wallace Foundation, an idea I had which George Lawrence has been helping me with. I set it up in 2005, and the idea is for me to become personally involved in helping to organise events such as golf days and dinners which I hope will bring in money. Having my own foundation means that I will retain control over the money and be able to direct it to various places where I believe it will be of most use to sufferers. Hopefully I can work with and alongside the MS Society, because they have so many different branches around the country and also have knowl-edge of where any funds we generate might be best used. I want to get much more involved with the MS Society. If I can go out, talk to people and maybe help them through some bad times, then I would like to do that. I also hope I will be able to raise public awareness of the illness.

On a personal level, things haven't been this good for me in ages. I'm happier now with my life than I have been at any time since I stopped playing football. My relationship with my children is also better now than it ever has been. I did have one final run-in with Remi around the time he was eighteen because I just felt he was let-ting his life pass him by. I basically told him to leave the house, which might sound a harsh thing to do, but I thought he needed a taste of reality. He went to live with his girlfriend Dianne, and in January 2003 they had a baby boy called Harlei. Unfortunately, Remi and Diane split up, and Remi now lives in London with his cousins, but at least we can talk to each other without a row developing. I love Remi and always will. I believe he knows that, and perhaps this book will help him to understand in some way how sorry I am that I didn't have a better relationship with him earlier in his life. Diane is a lovely girl, and Jen and I see her and Harlei regularly. She often comes round for Sunday lunch, and I love playing with my grandson. I just wish I'd done the same thing with his father. But I know I can't turn the clock back, and if there is one thing I have learnt since having MS, it is the importance of looking forward.

Elisha has been a lovely daughter to me. She enjoys football and loves watching John Terry play for Chelsea. We often sit together watching matches, and she will pipe up with questions about the game and about football in general. She's even prepared to watch old videos of me flying around the pitch with an afro haircut, or wearing a terrible sheepskin jacket when I'm being interviewed after a match. She's told me that she was proud of what I did and the fact that she is my daughter, but she can't be half as proud as I am to be her dad.

Thaila and I still seem to have the bond we built up during those early years, and I have a very easy-going and relaxed relationship with him. He's a lovely kid who helped me get through some difficult times simply by being there and making me realise I had something worth clinging on to. He probably didn't realise how important those times we had together were to me, but I hope he does now.

I also hope that Jenny realises she means everything to me. If it wasn't for her I don't think I would be here today. She has made sure that I have a life, and as long as she is beside me, it will always be a life worth living.

EPILOGUE

MARATHON TASK

I never shirked a challenge when I was playing football, and recently I have tried to bring that same philosophy back into my life. When you are told you have MS, life becomes much more of a challenge. For a long time I found myself unwilling to rise to it, but over the last few years I feel I've been getting to grips with the problems of my illness, just as other sufferers have to. It may have taken me some time, but I'm now at a point in my life where I feel I want to help others cope with the disease. One of the most practical ways of doing this is to raise money for the Multiple Sclerosis Society, and at the same time raise awareness of the condition so that the general public have a better understanding of what it is and what it does to individuals.

So when it was suggested that a good way of doing both would be for me to walk the London Marathon course, not only did it seem like a good idea, it also provided me with a huge challenge that really appealed. Once upon a time the thought of taking just a few steps in public brought me out in a cold sweat, but my confidence since that testimonial match at Southampton has really increased. Don't get me wrong, I'm still basically a shy person and I don't like drawing attention to myself, but my self-esteem has returned. I've also come to realise that the competitiveness that was always there as a player has never really left me. It may have been dormant for several years, but the idea of trying to complete a 26-mile marathon course was so attractive that it woke it up.

I had watched with real admiration in 2003 as former boxer Michael Watson, who so nearly lost his life following a brain operation he had to undergo after his fight with Chris Eubank in 1991, took on what appeared to be an impossible task and completed the marathon course in six days. Michael had to rebuild his whole life after that operation, and despite all the pain and the odds, which were stacked against him, he showed a true champion's spirit and desire to get across that finishing line and at the same time raise money and awareness for the Brain and Spine Foundation. It was an incredibly brave thing to do, and it was also inspirational.

A little over a year later I was asked if I fancied trying to do the same thing in aid of the MS Society. Geraldine Davies, who had been instrumental in sorting out and planning Michael's walk, got together with George Lawrence and the two of them started to lay plans for me to enter the 2005 marathon. I loved the idea of attempting the course, but unfortunately I hadn't thought much about the time and preparation needed. To put it simply, it became clear that I would need more of both if I was going to have a realistic chance of seeing the thing through, and in the end I decided not to enter that year. But the idea of undertaking the marathon really struck a chord with me, and I was sure that if I gave myself enough time to train properly I would have a better chance.

So in the autumn of 2005 I began preparing in earnest for a crack at the 2006 race. I knew that if I was going to do it I had to work gradually towards getting my mind and body conditioned for the task of walking four or five miles every day for six successive days. I knew it would be tough – even walking a few yards can be painful for me – but I was determined to give myself the best chance I could of completing the course, and in doing so raise funds for the Society. I started by taking short walks every day, and gradually built them up in time and length. Jenny also decided it would be useful for me to have a treadmill for when the weather started to get worse during the winter months, and I used it on a regular basis in order to increase my strength and stamina. After a few months of this, the difference in my overall fitness and body tone was amazing. The regime had a really good effect on me mentally as well, because I could feel myself getting fitter, and with that came greater confidence.

Not all days were good, of course. I had my setbacks, including one three-day period during which I just felt too weak to carry on with the training. But the overall feeling and effect it had on me was positive. My legs got stronger and I found it really exciting to be working towards an attempt at the 2006 London Marathon. In a funny way it was a bit like being a player again. I had to make sure I was fit for the game, and I had to be determined to rise to the challenge. I might not be in the same physical shape any more, but I soon began to realise that even getting myself in good enough condition to take part in the marathon would be an achievement I could be proud of for the rest of my life. Yes, I wanted to do it for selfish reasons – I knew it would give me something to aim for – but I also wanted to make sure that by getting involved I played a part in helping people with MS.

And that is something I intend to make sure I continue to do in the future, whether it's by raising money or awareness or both, or just being there to talk to fellow sufferers.

Although I have the illness, I feel lucky, because after all the dark times and agonies I went through I finally managed to get my life back, and it's a life I now feel comfortable with. I know I can never beat multiple sclerosis, but I can cope with it. If in the future in some small way I can help others to do the same, I will be delighted.

INDEX

INDEX